MW00356415

EAT
to CHEAT
DEMENTIA

What you eat helps avoid it or live better with it

by dietitian, Ngaire Hobbins
APD, BSc., Dip. Nutrition and Diet

First published in 2016

Margate, 7054, Hobart,
Tasmania

AUSTRALIA

Text © Ngaire Hobbins

Not to be copied in whole or in part without written authorisation.

ISBN 978-0-9943440-3-8

Design and book production Bermingham Books

Printed in Australia and globally through Ingram Spark

Contents

Introduction

If you have picked up this book, then dementia is a concern. Never forget that the vast majority of people currently living into their 70s, 80s, and 90s, *don't* have dementia and you can eat to boost your brain health to keep dementia at bay.

Not only that, but for anyone living with a diagnosis of dementia, food continues to hold the power to help you get the most out of each day, supporting brain and body, while continuing to add joy to life.

In my experience, the importance of eating and the disastrous consequences of the malnutrition that is all too common in dementia are frequently ignored. Often a flurry of tests and advice confront the recipient and those who care about them on diagnosis, so it's not surprising that the importance of eating can slip off the radar for the individual. Nevertheless, it is hard to believe that nutrition is also frequently overlooked by health care professionals and those working in dementia. Sure, if there has been significant weight loss or clearly poor food intake up to diagnosis, it might have become too obvious to ignore and measures put in place to deal with it. But sadly, by the time weight loss has progressed enough to become physically obvious to a casual observer, it can be exceedingly difficult to reverse it or reduce its impact.

My previous book *Eat To Cheat Ageing* looked in great detail at the damage weight loss does in later age and the disastrous effects of malnutrition, providing strategies for avoiding it and minimising it's impact in those for whom it is an issue. This is no less important when it comes to brain health as was recognised in 2014 in the report on nutrition and dementia by *Alzheimer's Disease International* (ADI) which states that close to half of those diagnosed with dementia had lost weight in the previous year, the consequences of which include increased frailty, falls, and death.

Eat To Cheat Dementia expands the discussion and investigates further the impact eating has on brain health and cognition, and how these affect the ability of someone living with dementia to get the nutrition they need. It provides a window into the very complex science of brain health and cognition for the everyday reader and provides advice and strategies to maximise brain health and cognition.

For those living with a diagnosis of dementia, its focus is firmly on cherishing and enjoying life. The sheer pleasure of sharing meals is part of that but also, age-appropriate eating maintains both physical and mental capacity, dementia or not.

Despite massive efforts worldwide, there is still no cure for dementia, so it remains a fatal illness. However, to focus on dementia as an incurable illness, is to do people living with dementia and those who care about them a disservice. Like anyone else, someone living with dementia deserves to enjoy every bit of the life they have ahead, and maintaining physical health along with supporting the brain with good food and activity is key in that.

As dementia is a progressive illness, there will come a time in its course when so many brain connections have been lost and brain cells have died that the process of eating and digesting food becomes too challenging, and care focussing on comfort must take the place of usual care. That includes the food and drinks offered, if any, and this is covered in the chapters ahead. Palliative care managed with empathy and compassion is a gift that allows an individual at the end of life and all their loved ones to honour the life and the passing when that life is done: dementia or not.

This book is firmly based in the science of nutrition and brain health but is written for the everyday reader. The science involved is significantly more complex than that presented in *Eat To Cheat Ageing* to be sure, but that's the nature of the beast when it comes to neuroscience. I hope I have managed to wrangle the scientific gobbledegook into words that are helpful and informative.

This book is for anyone interested in the latest research on how to reduce the risk of developing cognitive decline and dementia. There are so very many exciting and enticing claims and pseudo-science accessible on the internet for you to read. They aim to convince you to buy pills, potions, or powders, to have you rush out to buy the latest high Andean berry elixir, rid your cupboards of every morsel of familiar food now deemed the latest dietary evil, or to give up everyday foods you had previously thought were good for you. The fact is there is no miracle food or even a miracle diet, guaranteed to save you from dementia.

Unfortunately, many exciting claims for the latest 'super food', or revolutionary new diet, 'cherry pick' from the research, choosing what supports the case for the product being promoted.

In the face of that, the true science, which continues to support variety, moderation, and things that really do make sense when you can see the big picture, can pale into insignificance. My aim is to 'cut through the hype' as they say, give you the facts and the keys to make choices based on what we know now, that give your brain the best chance in the years ahead.

In the five or so years since I was researching to produce *Eat to Cheat Ageing,* it's been fantastic to see the huge boom in research on Alzheimer's disease and other dementias. When that book was conceived, there wasn't enough information for a whole book on dementia. We are so fortunate that there's been enough research carried out in this area that some things now accepted as fact were only theories just a few years ago.

This book is not about curing or even sure-fire ways to avoid dementia – there are none of those proven yet. It's about giving your brain the best chance you can to head off dementia if possible, or to help you live with it if you have had a diagnosis. There are three ways what you eat can assist in that – by helping keep your vascular system (blood vessels) running smoothly, by minimising the harmful effects wrought by inflammation and oxidative stress, and by eating foods that protect and support brain function.

We are living longer, so our bodies and brains have to endure the wear and tear of everyday life and function longer than the generations before ours needed them to. Maybe that's part of the reason we see more dementia. Certainly there are contributors in things over which we have limited control like our genes, injuries, and environmental influences, but we now have a wealth of information about minimising our own risk in the face of that and making the most of life even with a diagnosis of dementia.

However, no matter what our genes or our life up to today has presented, each of us has power to maximise our brain health.

That's what this book is about.

I do hope you enjoy.

Ngaire

Chapter 1

GETTING A HANDLE ON COGNITIVE DECLINE AND DEMENTIA

Dementia? Memory lapse? Cognitive decline? Or Alzheimer's?

I've thought a lot about what it might be like to experience dementia and spoken to people who are doing just that, and to me, living with dementia seems like navigating a very tricky maze. We negotiate mazes so often in our lives – whether that is dealing with a new social situation, solving a problem of study or work, or carrying out all the steps to prepare and enjoy a meal. As long as you have practiced a lot, it is easier and even if it's a new experience, if you lose your way you can bring in strategies you have used before to get you from the start to the end.

But in dementia, I think of it as being in a maze with added and changing challenges. In the early stages, the exit has been moved, making getting out a bigger challenge, but with time, perseverance, and bringing in strategies previously used in other situations in life, it can still be done. As the illness progresses however, the exit seems to move more frequently, adding to the challenges. Eventually, the walls of the maze also begin to move while you are in there – confusion increases and the chance of choosing the right path or getting out reduces. I don't know about you but I can see how confronting, even scary that could be. A caring friend could be standing at the exit calling, but if the walls have moved, you are now completely lost inside. What's needed are friends with maps and guiding hands to help.

With the idea of an increasingly complicated maze as a backdrop, let's begin to get a bit of a perspective on dementia – what it is, what it isn't – and some things you should watch out for before you worry that you have it. I'm not going to provide a lot of detail here into the different types of dementia and how many people get it, etc. – there are plenty of places you can find that information. My aim is to provide some keys to understanding what's going on and provide strategies to deal with that.

~ ~ ~

Always remember that poor memory, periods of confusion or even altered behaviour can be due to illness or stress, or just a result of the huge number of other things that you have going on in your brain the older you get.

~ ~ ~

The word *cognition* covers all the *thinking* processes of the brain: coordinating things like memory, language (both understanding it and speaking), insight and judgment, problem solving and decision-making. But even if you do find yourself with memory problems or have been diagnosed with mild cognitive impairment (or mild cognitive decline as it is also known), there is a lot you can still do to help your brain and to slow the possible progression to dementia.

First and foremost, don't delay in discussing any concerns with your GP or geriatrician. It's understandable to be anxious about receiving a diagnosis you don't want, but memory lapses and confusion can be caused by completely treatable conditions. If you put off mentioning these concerns to your doctor, you could miss your chance of having something treatable, dealt with quickly, so you can get back to enjoying life.

There are strategies and medications available, which can help delay the progression of cognitive decline and dementia, and there is an enormous amount of work being done to find more. If you delay that visit to your doctor then the benefits you might be able to get from these – especially anything brand new - will be reduced.

In addition, health practitioners are now increasingly aware that some medications prescribed to treat other conditions can affect the cognition of older people. This is particularly so when more than three different medications are being taken (this is called polypharmacy). Polypharmacy might contribute also to developing delirium.

If you go to your doctor as soon as you are aware of any symptoms that might be of concern, your current medications can be reviewed, and any that might be causing problems reconsidered. The great thing about checking that out too when it comes to eating well is that many medications also reduce appetite, and that is not something that is helpful in later age, and certainly not in most people with cognitive impairment or dementia. More on that later.

~ ~ ~

Is it dementia or just a temporary memory lapse?

Increasing forgetfulness doesn't necessarily mean dementia. In many cases, with practice, your memory can improve. Everyone has occasions when they can't remember where they've left the car keys, 'Why did I walk into this room?' or "What was I going to do?' moments.

Forgetfulness might even be a blessing; after all, if you remembered every person you met and every tiny thing that happened to you in your life, it would drive you crazy!

However, a little beyond forgetfulness is what's called cognitive decline or mild cognitive impairment. This is something that needs attention to give you the best chance of stopping it in its tracks or at least slowing it down. But no matter how qualified a health professional is, if they don't know you really well, detecting subtle changes can be hard. Most people are aware themselves, or have seen in a friend or family member things that just don't seem quite right. There are tell-tale signs:

- forgetting things more than now and then that would usually be remembered easily,
- struggling to find words or names for well-known people and things,
- consistently misplacing everyday things,
- losing the train of thought or the conversation thread repeatedly,
- finding it difficult to follow the plot in movies or books,
- feeling overwhelmed by making decisions, and
- making increasingly poor judgments in all sorts of situations.

These are the first and most important indicators that further investigation is warranted.

Cognitive decline can certainly be annoying but it doesn't overly interfere with your everyday life. It might show up on tests and be obvious to you and to others who know you well, but it's usually manageable and more often than not doesn't progress further. If you do regular exercise — both physical and mental — and eat appropriately, it can even improve.

Unfortunately, mild cognitive impairment for up to 20 percent of people will move on to dementia in a few years. It's when some or all of these cognitive abilities permanently decrease – affecting personality, appropriate interaction with the world around, and the capacity to carry out everyday tasks we usually take for granted like dressing, preparing meals or finding a way home - that it starts to become distressing.

This is when it's so important to seek professional assessment because tests can now be done that might identify not only things that could be fixed as mentioned before, but also to identify any signs of dementia that may be able to be treated to hold progression at bay. If there are signs that mild cognitive impairment is likely to move onto Alzheimer's or another form of dementia then it's possible to make plans for managing life in the years ahead so life with dementia remains enjoyable and fulfilling.

~ ~ ~

How does dementia or Alzheimer's disease differ from cognitive decline?

Dementia (including Alzheimer's disease which is by far the most common type affecting around 70% of those with dementia) is not a normal part of the ageing process and cognitive decline is only part of the picture. The types and their basic differences are outlined in the box here, but they all have something in common: all interfere with your everyday life and, therefore, often the lives of those around you.

Everyone with dementia is different. But when dementia throws up things like not being able to learn or remember new information, repeating stories or questions over and over, having difficulty finding words for familiar things, jumbling words and phrases, losing or hiding possessions, forgetting how or when to do everyday activities, making irrational or unusually poor financial decisions, becoming agitated and confused, and even suffering hallucinations, it requires understanding from caretakers, family members, and friends.

While dementia is a progressive, and at this stage remains a fatal illness, a diagnosis by no means implies that life is over there and then as so many people fear. On average, people have 10 to 14 years following diagnosis (though some will have 5 years and some up to 20). Having a good understanding of the disease, good management strategies, and sensible planning for dealing with progression of the illness means there is no reason why people with dementia cannot continue to live well for most of those years.

One thing that is far too often overlooked is a person's weight loss. Very many people lose weight in the months and years before a diagnosis of dementia is made, and many continue to do so following it. This is not useful weight loss designed to intentionally shed body fat, instead it's malnutrition and it has the power to snatch away quality of life, to further impact cognition, and hamper physical health. Watching out for weight loss and eating issues and developing strategies to address any problems as soon as possible, is extremely important in keeping pleasure in life as well as staying as well and healthy as possible. Unintentional weight loss in anyone above 70 is a risk factor for dementia as well as for physical decline and illness. We will get into this in detail later in this book.

However, before we go on, I want to touch on three things in particular that can masquerade as dementia: delirium, depression, and vitamin B12 deficiency. Some of the same traits you see gradually revealing themselves in dementia — confusion, agitation, disorientation, incoherent speech, unusual apathy, hallucinations, and extremes of emotion — can also be caused by delirium, and some by a deficiency of vitamin B12. Depression in an older person can produce apathy, unresponsiveness, and apparent inability to communicate so it can also look like dementia. The very big difference is, unlike dementia, depression, delirium, and B12 deficiency are reversible, and treating B12 deficiency completely removes those symptoms when done promptly. Delirium and late life depression can be risk factors for subsequent dementia but treating them as soon as possible also reduces the chance it will develop.

~ ~ ~

Delirium

Delirium is a serious, life threatening medical condition that can occur when you have an infection, experience fever, after a general anaesthetic (this is very common in older people), when you are dehydrated, and in a number of illnesses.

It's 'red herrings' like confusion, disorientation, apathy, and hallucinations that can make diagnosis very tricky at times. A delirium might look like dementia to the casual observer; it's easy to suspect it as the culprit when there's no obvious illness or fever. Nevertheless, there is an important clue to diagnosing it: delirium usually comes on quickly and the symptoms can come and go, even with a day or so in between at times, though usually more pronounced at night. Dementia, in contrast, usually develops gradually over weeks, months, or years and, once evident, symptoms tend to be constant.

You'd think it would be obvious if a delirium were due to an infection or similar because there'd be pain or fever but if you are already taking medication to control pain elsewhere in the body then the tell-tale signs can easily be masked.

Common medications taken for chronic pain will also reduce fever and of course counter any sort of pain – not just that in your knees or lower back for example – so a delirium can be developing from an infection you don't even feel the effects of. It's actually common for infections bubbling away deep under your teeth, in your urinary tract, or even in your lungs, to cause no pain or obvious illness to alert you to their presence.

In older age also, a number of changes in body systems alter the sensing of thirst, so dehydration becomes more likely and it's quite possible to be unaware of it. Dehydration is a common cause of delirium at all ages but much more so in later age.

In yet another annoying reality, the older you get, the more likely you are to suffer a delirium during an illness, particularly if you regularly take more than four different medications of any kind, or if you have Parkinson's disease, already have dementia, or have previously had a stroke. Moreover, if it happens once, there is a high chance, unfortunately, that it will happen again.

As mentioned above, remember that medications themselves can cause delirium; you may not tolerate a new medication prescribed for you, or you might accidentally take more of one than you should. Sometimes there is an interaction between different medications and sometimes you may have done well on a particular dosage level for many years but changes in the way your body deals with it as you age mean side effects can surface. One of those can be delirium.

The message is that any sudden change in someone's usual behaviour needs a visit to the doctor. And before you even think about changing anything yourself, you must not stop taking any prescribed medication without first discussing any concerns you have with your doctor. The sudden change itself might trigger delirium or cause other health issues. Have a look at the list in the box below. If you have any concerns, your doctor can organise a thorough review of your medications — something that should always be done anyway if you have experienced delirium.

Delirium is usually a sign of other undiagnosed problems that need treatment to stop them doing more damage. If you do suffer delirium there's also more chance your illness will put you in the hospital, so unless you are planning that relaxing experience, it's best to consult your doctor quickly.

SOME OF THE MEDICATIONS THAT MAY TRIGGER DELIRIUM IN OLDER AGE

NOTE: DO NOT STOP TAKING MEDICATIONS PRESCRIBED FOR YOU WITHOUT CHECKING FIRST WITH YOUR DOCTOR. DOING SO COULD CAUSE SERIOUS HARM.

All medications are prescribed for specific reasons and most people don't have any problem with them or, if they do, the side effects should quickly diminish. With advancing age and increasing medical issues, problems may occur with some medications on this list. If you are concerned at all for yourself or someone you care for, then discuss your options with your doctor as soon as possible. The list is only a guide and includes common brand names. Generic brands of some medications and those released recently may not be listed here.

Common brand names in Australia are shown in italics

Heart medications:	digoxin (*Lanoxin*) and disopyramide (*Rythmodan*) — both anti-arrhythmia drugs; isosorbide (*Isordil, Isogen, Imdur, Monodur, Sorbidin, Iimtrate*) for angina
Blood pressure drugs:	nifedipine (*Adalat, Adapine, Nifecard, Adefin*). This medication is also used for angina and Raynaud's disease
Anti-Parkinson's medications:	levodopa (*Madopar, Sinemet, Kinson*)
Fluid tablets:	frusemide (*Lasix, Urex*)
Sedatives:	Barbiturates (*Phenobarbitone, Amylobarbitone*) benzodiazepines (including *Xanax, Kalma, Valium, Serepax, Ativan, Diazepam, Rivotril, Murelax*) alcohol
Anti-epileptic/ anti-psychotic medications:	phenytoin (*Dilantin*)
Some antidepressants:	lithium (*Lithicarb, Quilonium*), SSRIs (including *Zoloft, Aropax, Cipramil, Lexapro, Prozac, Lovan*) and TCAs (tricyclic antidepressants, including *Tryptanol, Allegron, Endep, Tolerade, Tofranil*)

Opioids (for strong pain):	codeine (marketed as *Codeine*, also *Aspalgin, Codis, Codral, Codalgin, Mersyndol*, and in many cold and flu medications), morphine (*Anamorph, MS Contin, MS Mono, Kapanol*), oxycodone (*Endone, Oxynorm, Oxycontin*), tramadol (*Tramal*) and pethidine (*Parnate, Nardil*)
Some NSAIDS (non-steroidal anti-inflammatories, for pain and inflammation):	including ibuprophen (*Nurofen* and many generics) and naproxen (*Naprosyn*), available *over the counter* and a number of common prescription NSAIDs:, diclofenac (*Voltaren*), celecoxib (*Celebrex*), meloxicam (*Mobic*), piroxicam (*Feldene*), indomethacin (*Indocid*), mefanamic acid (*Ponstan*)
Some anti-ulcer drugs:	cimetidine (*Tagamet*)
A corticosteroid:	Prednisone (*Delta-cortef, Panafcortelone, Solone, Premix, Sterofrin, Prednefrin forte, Panafcort, Sone, Medrol*)
Antihistamine:	promethazine (*Phenergan, Painstop syrup, Prothazine, Panquil, Seda-quell, Avomine, Tixylix*). These are older type antihistamines — the ones that also tend to cause drowsiness.
Some antibiotics:	quinolones (including *Ciproxin, Avelox, Noroxin*) penicillin-related drugs amoxycillin (including *Amoxil, Moxacin, Cilamox, Alphamox, Fisamox, Augmentin, Clavulin*) and flucloxacillin (including *Floxapen, Flopen, Flucil, Staphylex*), the cephalosporins (including *Keflex, Ceporex, Ibilex, Ceclor, Keflor*)

~ ~ ~

Depression

Depression can in fact be a part of dementia, but it's always worth seeking advice because if it's not dementia then treating it can put the person back on track. If it is dementia, nothing has been lost in checking.

~ ~ ~

B12 deficiency

A deficiency of vitamin B12 also causes confusion and memory problems and it's something that can be too easily mistaken for dementia. But B12 deficiency is easily detected with a simple blood test and then is completely reversible if treated promptly. Delaying treatment, on the other hand, can cause permanent damage to your brain and nervous system. You can read more on this vitamin in Chapter 4.

~ ~ ~

How the brain should work, and what happens when dementia makes things go wrong

Getting a basic understanding of the way dementia might be affecting the normal working of the brain can make living with and understanding dementia just a bit less challenging. Without that, it can be very hard not to take things personally if you live with someone who seems to be doing things just to make your life more difficult or behaving in ways they never have before. And if you are living with dementia yourself in its early stages, it can help make sense of some of the things you are experiencing.

The brain is made up of a number of different parts that have distinct functions – How a dementia plays out depends on what parts are damaged and that varies with the type of dementia. By far the largest part of the brain is the cerebral cortex, which is made up of four lobes. The frontal lobe is mostly where personality lies and it handles speech, mood, thinking, planning and skilled motor activity. The temporal lobe is involved with hearing, some language skills, perception, emotion, judgement, and memory. The parietal lobe integrates complex sensory information from the body and contributes to the understanding of language. The occipital lobe is mostly involved with vision. There is also the cerebellum at the lower rear of the cortex, which does an enormous amount of the housekeeping in the body and maintains balance and muscle activity. The brain stem is predominantly involved in transferring information to and from the brain and the body. Last but not least, the hippocampus, lying deep inside the folds of the cortex, has vital roles in memory – in particular short-term memory.

To do all the things the brain needs to do every second of every day, individual nerves (neurones) communicate between themselves, passing messages via chemicals called neurotransmitters from neurones inside and outside the brain, connecting in the brain and sending responses back via neurones to the rest of the body.

Anything that stops the transmissions between neurones – be it a blockage between cells, problems within a cell, or the unavailability of the right neurotransmitter –means that messages can't get through. Add to that the impact of any interruption to the supply of resources the neurones need and the ability to get rid of things they don't need and problems are exacerbated.

Think for a moment of the complexities involved in answering a simple question: "Would you like tea or coffee?" That sound needs to be directed to the right place in the brain, interpreted to give it meaning and context, and then an appropriate response needs to be concocted. That is done by weaving in memories, feelings, and thirst levels, and then muscles need to be instructed to make the right combination of sounds at the appropriate volume and tone to relay all that in order to get the drink.

If there is a hiccup in any of those steps things go awry. If the response to the question is accidentally "Where is the car?" or if instead the person gets up and wanders off, it doesn't necessarily mean they wouldn't like a cup of tea, it could be the connections have been jumbled. Too often in fact, people go hungry or thirsty for just those reasons.

Think too of reading – those are merely pen marks on paper or scribbles on a screen unless a complex interaction of memories from school days and more recent experience combine with the context (a menu? a book? a label on a medication? an instruction manual? a post on Facebook?) and more to interpret them.

And then there is food. To eat it's necessary to access ingredients for meals and that could involve driving, negotiating supermarket aisles and/or communicating with shopkeepers, and then making it home again with the items. Then there are recipes to remember or to decipher and follow, ovens, stoves, or barbecues to manage, plating up and cutlery to help get it in. It's no wonder it can get challenging to eat if the maze exit keeps moving, as might seem to be the case if for example, the stove has become inexplicable or cutlery confusing.

Many people who have lived full lives and managed complex problems at work before their diagnosis are able to cover up issues for quite some time. They achieve this by bringing in other strategies and that may explain to some extent why some, when diagnosed, are actually more progressed in the disease than others are.

As dementia progresses, more connections are lost and eventually neurones die, and with that progressively increasing damage goes ability.

It's important to be aware that a person living with dementia – especially in the earlier stages when they are mostly functioning quite well and problems may not be obvious to people who don't know them well - is probably even more frustrated than an observer in situations where this confusion of messaging is happening, so patience and empathy are always important.

~ ~ ~

Life gives the brain more than just keeping us functioning in our world. Every new experience, every challenge mastered, every skill practiced and honed, all the ways we dare our brains to do new things forces it to set up more and more complex internal networks –making more and more connections between individual cells. This is what's called cognitive reserve and it's rather like a road access into a small town. If there is only a single road in and out of town and the bridge over the river on that road is destroyed by flood, traffic flow is going to stop completely. If there is an alternate route up over the hill then it's possible to get to town but things will slow up a bit. But if there is a network of roads in the area then it's just a matter of using an alternate route to get where you need to go. The more experience the brain gets, the bigger the network of connections – the cognitive reserve - it develops and the more chance that it will be able to use alternate routes to continue carrying out complex tasks for many years.

A greater cognitive reserve provides the brain with more space to adapt if connections are lost at one point or other. The more experience you can give your brain at any age, both physically and mentally, the better chance you have of weathering any such problems later on, should they occur.

And what's interesting is that despite most people in their 80s and 90s probably having at least some evidence of the amyloid plaques that are associated with Alzheimer's disease, and some patches of damage from blood flow interruptions (called ischaemic damage), not everyone gets Alzheimer's disease or other dementias. Even those who do have plaque or ischaemic damage may still live many years longer without evidence of dementia. It may be that having a greater cognitive reserve when you hit your later years is part of that.

SOME COMMON TESTS USED TO DETERMINE COGNITIVE CAPACITY

Mini-Mental Status Examination (MMSE)

This is the most common test for the screening of dementia. It assesses skills such as reading, writing, orientation, and short-term memory.

Alzheimer's Disease Assessment Scale-Cognitive (ADAS-Cog)

This is more thorough than the MMSE and is more often used for people with mild symptoms.

It is a good examination especially for memory and language skills.

Neuropsychological Testing

This involves a more comprehensive series of tests usually administered by a neuropsychologist (a psychologist specialist dealing with dementia and other disorders of the brain).

SOME PATHOLOGY TESTS

Some pathology tests that might be used to check for cognitive decline or dementia and what they are looking for

Amyloid deposition

CSF - test for reduced levels β amyloid in CSF (cerebrospinal fluid): implies possible accumulation in the brain

PET imaging: detects β amyloid in the brain by PET scan

Neurodegeneration

CSF – detects changes in tau protein type and/or amount in CSF

MRI – checks changes in the volume of the hippocampus by MRI scan

Brain PET scan – checks for reduced glucose utilisation in the brain

A RUN-DOWN ON SOME COMMON TYPES OF DEMENTIA

Type of dementia	about	Common aspects
Alzheimer's dementia (AD)	Around 70% of all cases of dementia Affects 1 in 4 people over 85 Generalised atrophy, especially in the medial/temporal areas	Short term memory difficulties Vagueness in everyday conversation Seeming loss of enthusiasm for previously enjoyed activities Increased time taken to do routine tasks Forgetting well-known people or places Apparent inability to understand questions or carry out instructions Deterioration of social skills Emotional unpredictability Making increasingly poor judgements Reduced empathy and insight
Vascular Dementia	20-30% A broad term for any reduction in cognition resulting from restricted blood flow in the brain Tends to increase as additional events reducing blood flow occur.	Symptoms depend on brain area affected and can include any listed here in other types of dementia. Symptoms may be greater soon after a TIA or similar (temporary blockage of blood flow) and can improve at least temporarily but then worsen with reoccurrence.
Lewy body dementia	Two forms – Parkinson's dementia and dementia with lewy bodies Therapy is able to reduce symptoms in some people at least for a time.	Symptoms vary but can include: Visual hallucinations Behavioural and mood disorders Sleep issues (extreme activity during sleep can occur) Tremor or slowed walking Fluctuating alertness or cognition

| frontotemporal dementia (FTD) | Much less common than other forms of dementia but tends to affect younger people (45 to 60yrs) | Three types (behavioural, semantic, progressive fluent) but behavioural is the most common.

Symptoms include:

Poor judgement of right and wrong, moral or immoral, and safe or unsafe.

Loss of inhibition leading to inappropriate behaviour.

Poor judgement in finances and complex decisions.

Loss of interest in people and loss of empathy. |

Chapter 2

RESOURCING THE BRAIN

What a brain needs

Your brain needs a few resources to do the myriad of tasks we ask of it each day – it needs a variety of substances, called neurotransmitters, to help its cells speak to each other and the rest of the body. It also needs fuel, water, and particular nutrients supplied where and when they are needed, so it can achieve what you expect of it.

In the next chapter, we will look at specific micronutrient resources in detail, and especially how you can easily eat foods that will help your brain. Here I want to look at a bigger picture: how the brain runs, how it is protected, how it's fuelled and hydrated, and how what you do every day through practice, activity, and the way you live can help it stay healthy.

Don't panic – we are not doing neuroscience 101 here; there are just a few things that are worth knowing before we go into helping the brain out. Firstly, the brain has extremely good defence systems in place. That makes sense, it being so important to everything we do, but it has also made it very challenging in research, because those defences have stopped scientists getting a good look inside it for centuries. So recent advances in medical technology that have allowed researchers to get a clearer picture of many things that were only guessed about before, are all the more exciting. A lot of what we now know about dementia is a result of that, and there will be much more to come.

~ ~ ~

One thing that we have known about for a long while is the blood brain barrier. This protective barrier only allows some substances through to the neurones (or nerve cells) in the brain. It is also the reason why some things that neurones might need and many medications can't get in easily. Some substances like glucose get across with the assistance of specialised carriers and if they are in short supply or not working effectively, glucose can't get to where it's needed to carry out the tasks it is destined to do.

The neurones speak to each other and to other nerves coming in from the body and going away from the brain by means of neurotransmitter chemicals. These are produced in the neurones and act as messengers over the gaps between them. Additionally, there are a huge number of support cells: these are called glia collectively but you might also hear astrocytes or microglia being mentioned, and there are 10 to 50 times as many of these as neurones in the brain. They provide nourishment and support for neurones, clean up waste and damaged cells, and possibly assist with blood flow and fuel supply, as you will read later.

The brain loves working and the more it does in learning and carrying out tasks and activities, the more connections are made between various neurones. Training and practice keeps those active and builds extra cells and connections as needed. The brain relishes activity, is even able to *rewire* if connections are severed or damaged for any reason by injury or trauma; that rewiring ability is called plasticity, and gives it some flexibility to adapt. To make these new connections and maintain plasticity the brain relies on a number of chemicals, including brain derived neurotrophic factor or BDNF (something the brain makes that helps it to grow new neurones).

This highly complex and sensitive system deserves the very best protection available to keep it running smoothly. Cognitive decline and dementia are mostly the result of inadequacies in, or a failure of that protection.

Your genes may play a part but as is often quoted by researchers, "Genes load the gun, environment pulls the trigger." Even if you have the genes that increase your chance of dementia, you are like anyone else when it comes to doing what you can to help reduce that chance.

All brain cell activities produce waste products that can be damaging. However, damage control is managed by delicately balanced systems within the cells. The accumulation of β amyloid (or Beta Amyloid) into 'plaques', and the alteration of tau protein to form 'tangles' that are seen in Alzheimer's disease, are influenced by this balance. The 'plaques' and 'tangles' disrupt, or sever communication between neurones. Despite massive amounts of research having been done to try to work out how and why this happens, so far the answer has evaded us.

But there have been exciting breakthroughs - one just recently: it's been known for years that the cerebrospinal fluid bathing the brain was able to remove some of the waste of brain activity. However, the brain is so metabolically active it produces far more potentially harmful things than that system could possibly handle. Yet most people maintain good brain health. Therefore, scientists have been convinced that there had to be something else at work and it's only very recently that it was finally discovered. Technological advances now allow researchers to investigate the brain while it's actually working and they have revealed the incredible 'glymphatic system.'

This labyrinth of minute tubes throughout the brain actively pumps fluid to collect waste products gathered up by the glia, and move them out of the brain before they can do harm. What is extra interesting is that it seems it's while you are sleeping that it really swings into action more than during the day.

So there is more to sleep than just catching up on rest, it also gives your brain a chance to do a bit of an essential clear out. It may be that inefficient sleep over the years then could be part of the picture in dementia. It does make sense: any activity – be it body or brain, physical or mental – always needs to be balanced by rest.

It's worth mentioning while thinking about sleep that the brain can't achieve what it does – awake or sleeping – without an efficient supply of oxygen, and that is hampered during sleep, by sleep apnoea. This is a condition that reduces the amount of oxygen getting into the blood and therefore to the brain due to your breathing stopping intermittently during sleep. It's usually associated with snoring; and has recently been found to be linked with development of cognitive impairment and dementia.

Sleep apnoea is more common in people who are overweight or obese, and in those who smoke or snore. Interestingly, the glymphatic system is also thought to work best when you are sleeping on your side, so it's worth sticking to that position if it's your usual or using strategies to avoid sleeping on your back if you usually do. Those of you who snore might do well to get that checked out to avoid the possible damage sleep apnoea could do.

In people living with dementia, sleep can be an issue in itself because dementia can so often disrupt usual sleep patterns. People are awake when they usually wouldn't be and often fall asleep throughout the day when most are active– sleep apnoea may be part of that, but it's likely that these changed patterns are more a result of damage to parts of the brain that regulate sleeping and waking. The erratic sleep patterns in people with Alzheimer's disease are common, and possibly contribute to the progress of the dementia; and what is as much an issue, often significantly impact the lives of family members and caretakers.

As with most things discussed in this book, activity and exercise are key; physical activity encourages better sleep, so it helps your brain protect itself.

Along with sleep itself, there is a likely benefit from short periods of 'thought fasting' while awake that are a bit like the benefits that short eating fasts provide the body in younger people. What I mean is, giving the brain the opportunity to 'switch off' for periods of time. Whether that be through practicing meditation if that's your thing, or if not, anything that allows it to be 'quiet', like sitting in a park contemplating the view, spending time gazing at clouds, the ocean, or the expanse of a wide open vista, raking leaves or sweeping, tending a garden patch, or even washing dishes. Anything that allows you to focus peacefully on one simple task helps.

People who live long and well, maintaining healthy brains are known to engage in meditative practice regularly within their daily physically active lives. As our lives become increasingly busy, often filled with gadgets and devices designed to supply us with constant information and entertainment, it's increasingly important to find ways to give your brain a break now and then – including both good sleep and whichever way you choose, to allow it a 'switch off' time.

~ ~ ~

Maintenance and Logistics – the true meaning of 'lifeblood'

We've looked at the systems the brain has to protect and resource itself internally, but resources must come in from the body and what is not needed or is left over after it's done its work must be removed to keep it healthy. So a smooth and efficient logistics operation via the blood is essential. Anything that restricts blood flow to or through the brain, even in a small way, means less oxygen, fuel, and nutrients to work with and more accumulation of waste.

Complete blockage of blood supply can cause death of brain cells as happens in stroke and brain injury. Moreover, if blood is not flowing, neither can that fantastic glymphatic system, so harmful waste products get the chance to build up around and inside neurones. However, the effects of temporary or partial restriction to blood flow over many years are now thought to be part of the picture of dementia. A single instance of cell resources being reduced and toxic waste products allowed to hang around brain cells longer than they should is probably of little consequence, but over decades if those instances are repeated, the effects just might add up.

TIAs (transient ischaemic attacks) are part of that. These are also called *mini strokes* and happen when blood flow to an area of the brain is cut off or reduced temporarily, causing symptoms including the following:

- sudden weakness, numbness or paralysis in the face, arm(s) or leg(s),
- difficulty speaking or understanding,
- dizziness, loss of balance or an unexplained fall,
- a temporary loss of vision or suddenly having blurred or decreased vision in one or both eyes,
- difficulty swallowing or a sudden severe or unusual headache.

These experiences may disappear in a few minutes or stick around less than a day so it's common for them to be discounted or ignored. That is a bad idea because they might just be caused by things that can be treated like a migraine or an epileptic event. If not, they tend to keep happening if nothing is done and it's then that damage accumulates.

They can also be a warning of a 'real' stroke on the horizon and that is certainly something you'll want to avoid. If you get any of these symptoms, get yourself to the doctor to have them properly checked out.

~ ~ ~

Anything that contributes to changes in blood flow, or to increasing your risk of stroke such as elevated cholesterol or obesity in early or middle adulthood, needs attention for your brain's sake also. But be very aware that these need to be dealt with before you reach older age. Mid-life obesity is certainly associated with an increased chance of dementia in later age and high cholesterol is a significant risk factor for heart attack and stroke as well as cognitive problems – but once you are in your late 70s and beyond the situation with losing weight is different. This is covered in much greater detail in *Eat To Cheat Ageing* but suffice to say, dieting to lose weight in later age often does more harm than good and cholesterol may need to be handled differently, so if you are concerned read more in that book.

~ ~ ~

It's worth remembering that your brain is highly vulnerable to the effects of either high or low blood pressure so keeping it within healthy limits is also important. If your blood pressure is consistently higher than it should be, that can damage tiny blood vessels in the brain, starving areas of resources and even causing cell death. That's why your doctor regularly monitors your blood pressure and it's especially important as you age because blood vessels lose their elasticity as time goes on, just like your skin and that makes it harder to pump blood efficiently. But unlike your skin, it's possible to keep up elasticity in blood vessels through exercise, at least in part. The actions of muscles during activity help blood move around to provide an extra helping hand.

~ ~ ~

Low blood pressure is not as widely discussed as high but in older people, it can present problems for the brain. One thing that is quite common in is called postural hypotension – that's medical gobbledegook for low blood pressure that happens when you stand up quickly. When this happens, the brain temporarily doesn't get the blood flow it needs, causing dizziness, light-headedness, and falls so it's something to be avoided. But apart from the danger it presents by causing a calamitous fall, it also means the brain isn't getting the oxygen it needs at that time because blood flow is temporarily reduced, and that can certainly add up to create permanent damage and cognitive issues if not addressed.

~ ~ ~

CELL DAMAGE AND BLOOD FLOW RESTRICTION: CHICKEN OR EGG IN THE DEVELOPMENT OF DEMENTIA?

At any point in time a large part of your brain is doing day to day tasks like keeping you breathing, keeping your heart beating, and organs doing what they do– the sort of things you don't want to waste time thinking about, but without which you wouldn't be alive. These tasks use about the same amount of resources and produce the same amount of waste day in day out so the amount of blood moving through these areas doesn't need to fluctuate dramatically to keep them up to scratch. But that's not the case for the cognitive powerhouse of the brain in the cerebral cortex. This is where planning and thinking activity is done, where your personality lies, where all complex thought processes are managed and the place where dementia first shows its cards.

While this part of the brain is never 'silent', it can be 'quiet' during sleep for example, but revs up dramatically when you are trying to sort problems, do your finances, crosswords or Sudoku, read a book, play tennis, drive a car, learn something new or anything that requires integration of many variables, complex thought and and/or planning. Unless the supply and clear-up systems also rev up dramatically to keep pace, none of these things will be able to be maintained for long and brain health will suffer.

It's only recently that technological advances have let us look into the working brain to discover that the glia produce messenger substances bringing about dramatic increases in blood flow in the area of the brain doing the extra work.

But glia affected by inflammation and oxidative stress may not be able to do that efficiently. As a result the chances of ramping up blood flow to active areas is reduced, neurones can't achieve what they need to and there is a much greater chance that further cell damage will occur, including the build-up of 'plaques' and 'tangles.' All this can happen well before any cognitive decline is evident.

So which does come first – cell damage or reduced blood flow and accumulation of toxic wastes?

We just don't know.

But whatever the starting point, it's likely a vicious cycle is set up of damage and further restriction of blood flow that must eventually affect the brain's ability to carry out complex tasks.

The root cause however most likely lies in inflammation and/or oxidative stress and even though we don't know yet exactly how it plays out, in practical terms that doesn't really matter: your best chance at prevention, probably lies again in ensuring you get plenty of antioxidants, eat well, and stay active.

~ ~ ~

Modern life, the overactive immune system, and the brain

Inflammation is the normal response to anything the body's defence systems deems to be harmful. It's an essential part of the immune response designed to fight off illness and infection. It helps set up for and manage any repair work that's needed if damage has occurred. And because the 'attack' can happen anywhere in the body the system employs an array of communicator chemicals that can gather assistance from wide and far to deal with the 'invader'. These chemicals do a fabulous job when there is an active threat to be dealt with, activating many body systems and orchestrating redirection of resources as needed - but unfortunately, too often the system doesn't switch off as it should when the threat has ceased and sometimes it starts up without a real threat having occurred.

This situation – called chronic inflammation - unfortunately happens a lot in our modern lives. In Eat To Cheat Ageing I discussed how this contributes to a loss of vital muscle tissue but also, it plays a part in the development of dementia.

Chronic inflammation is a bit like sitting in your car when it's stationary with the engine on and your foot on the accelerator - you are not going anywhere but you force the engine to use extra fuel, oil, and water, and to pump out exhaust when it could be idling or switched off. In chronic inflammation, cells are always switched on and are working 'uselessly'. They are using extra resources and producing extra toxic wastes but with the system chronically inflamed, the usual clean up systems to deal with these wastes are not given their usual priority. The consequence for the brain eventually is 'exhaustion' in some areas and build-up of substances like β amyloid. Inflammation is thought by many researchers to be the biggest challenge to our health as we age for these reasons as well as its effects elsewhere in the body.

So why does this happen? We don't have complete answers yet but many things we know play a part and we can easily work with them to increase our own chance of keeping inflammation under control.

Inactivity and lack of regular exercise are big contributors. Medical research shows that living a sedentary lifestyle is associated with a reduced brain volume and that increasing the activity levels of previously sedentary people reduces inflammatory activity. Therefore, exercise wins again - increasing the chance of maintaining good brain function.

The other thing research has shown is that there is just too much food available to most of us living in western society. It's not just obesity in young or middle adulthood that is the issue here; it's that regularly eating more food than your body needs each day (even if you don't get fat from that) triggers inflammation in itself. That is made worse if obesity is also part of the picture.

But take care again to consider your stage of life when you think about this. Avoiding chronic over consumption in younger and middle age is where the benefit lies – it's about eating meals as needed and not giving in to the constant food marketing that seems to suggest every waking moment needs to involve putting something in your mouth. No matter how *healthy* some foods are, adding them to an already complete day's meals might do more harm than good.

When you are past middle age the best thing to do is boost your activity levels in any way you can (or keep them up if you are already doing that) because that's a sure fire way to do your body a favour. Exercise in itself reduces inflammation in body and brain.

As you advance in age you need to be sure to keep up your nutrition, remembering that you need the same amount of most nutrients and extra of some including protein so you must not let your food intake dwindle. Dieting for weight loss at later age is not a good idea but boosting exercise and doing muscle activity will always be of more help in combating inflammation than anything else.

When it comes to eating to prevent inflammation, the same foods that protect from oxidative stress come out on top in protection against inflammation. Many of the substances you know as antioxidants and that are listed in the text box on page 31 are also able to combat excessive inflammation. Some, including flavonoids, resveratrol and others, have antioxidant actions throughout the body but also can move across the blood brain barrier where they have important neuroprotective and anti-inflammatory roles. Additionally, a number of foods supply substances known to reduce inflammation and protect cells – these include oily fish for its omega 3 fats; nuts, seeds and avocados for their monounsaturated fats and fibre; beans and legumes for their fibre and other important substances; and the oil from olives, nuts, and seeds. With all oils, but especially olive oil, choose the ones that have undergone the fewest steps in their production: extra virgin olive oil contains antioxidants as well as protective compounds that are removed with further refining.

The best advice is to try to eat foods that remain as close as possible to the way they came off the land, from the animal, or the sea. Foods that are commercially processed, specifically if that involves heating or cooking at high temperatures, especially repeatedly and/or adding extra fats, sugars, or salts, tend to increase inflammation. Deep fried or baked foods that are also high in salt and/or sugar, including many prominent takeaway foods are possible culprits too.

That doesn't mean never enter a supermarket or eat 'fast food' again – for most people they provide a convenient, accessible source of nutritious food. But as much as possible stick mostly to the fresh foods – vegetables, fruits, meat, fish, dairy, nuts, seeds, and legumes along with the good oil.

~ ~ ~

Modern life, oxidative stress and the brain

Oxidation is the process that every one of your body cells uses to carry out its unique function. Oxidation is absolutely essential to life, but it also results in waste products that you might know as 'free radicals', oxidants, or oxidative waste. They must be removed as soon as possible from within and around cells to avoid causing harm. This is especially important in your brain because its immense workload and capacity means that more oxidation happens there than in any other organ in your body. As we live longer, the accumulation of even tiny amounts of damage left behind, if oxidative wastes are not cleaned up, can eventually swamp your brain's ability.

Scientists have recently come to believe that β amyloid accumulation might start as a part of the brain's attempt at self-protection in the face of oxidative stress (a situation when oxidative damage is accumulating). But something goes wrong. Instead of providing that protection and then being removed when it's done, it instead accumulates, forming disruptive plaques and eventually impacts cognitive functions. It may be that the glia are part of what goes wrong, by not being able to help remove excess β amyloid when they are affected by inflammation and oxidative stress.

It also seems that oxidative damage messes up the ability of brain cells to use glucose properly and disrupts the workings of the mitochondria, which are the cells' power suppliers. The process becomes self-perpetuating because mitochondria that have suffered oxidative damage then produce more oxidative waste, thereby adding to oxidative stress.

It's a bit like a poorly maintained car. As the oil becomes degraded and dirty with repeated heating and cooling and extended use, and as tiny fragments of metal and plastics from inside gaskets and cylinders accumulate in the engine, its efficiency reduces so it uses more fuel, blows out more smoke and generally loses power. If maintenance continues to be neglected, fuel needs will increase, wastes accumulate, and things get progressively worse. Chances are it will just stop one day if this goes on long enough.

There is evidence that some people might be more susceptible to oxidative stress (and maybe inflammation) than others so their chances of developing Alzheimer's and other dementias are increased.

This probably (at least partly) comes down to an individual's genetic makeup, and while our understanding of the part that plays continues to grow and will assist in solving the puzzle in time, it's outside the scope of this book.

No matter what is found however, everyone can access the benefits of the protection against oxidative damage that comes from the myriad of fabulous and easily accessible substances that act as antioxidants. These mop up or neutralise oxidative wastes before they can wreak havoc. The more antioxidants you eat, the better chance you give your brain (as well as the rest of your body).

Antioxidants, and related food components go by a mystifying assortment of chemical names and some are also vitamins and essential minerals but, in a delightfully convenient twist of nature, different ones also happen to come from different coloured foods. So you really don't need to know much about nutrition to make sure you get plenty of antioxidants, you just need to eat a variety of colours. Ideally, eat at least five or six different coloured foods, or shades of colour at each meal, more if you can manage it.

Many intensely coloured foods are well known sources of antioxidants: think berries, cherries, red apples, egg yolk, dark green vegetables, green herbs, black olives, multi-coloured lettuce, black and green tea, turmeric and other spices, and the wide array of coloured fruits and vegetables, not to mention dark chocolate and red wine! But even paler foods like green and gold apples (both the flesh and the skin), nuts, fish, and mushrooms are good sources. You don't need much of each different food; you just need to think variety.

Some of these foods (especially walnuts, flax seeds and flax seed oil, canola oil) also provide the plant based Omega 3 fat ALA (alpha-linolenic acid) that plays a part in keeping blood vessels healthy, so benefits both the heart and the brain. Again, it's not huge amounts of any one food that does the job, it's eating as many different things as you can every day and every week, and reaping the many benefits that brings.

It's when the variety of foods you eat dwindles that your antioxidant intake also falls. Then it may be tempting to look towards the almost endless variety of commercial antioxidant supplements, drinks, and tablets on the market. Advertising claims can be seductive, convincing you that the latest berry or strange looking fruit from the high Himalayas or 'deepest darkest Peru' has the secret antioxidant to override all others. But the science is clear: it's the combination of many different antioxidants that give the best protection. And it seems that getting them from foods has the advantage. They may not work as effectively alone as they do when they are in the food they originally came from. There are other substances in the same foods that help in ways we are only just starting to understand and no doubt, more will be known of these in the next few years. What's important is realising that they are sociable little fellows, much happier working with the team they already know. We just can't be sure they are going to have the same impact when expected to work independently. Eating as many different coloured foods as possible is likely to be far more useful and it's easy to remember – such an advantage when every one of us worries our memories aren't what they once were!!

Unfortunately, the jury is out on whether they are able to reverse any damage already done, but one great thing is, that as long as food is your source of antioxidants and other vital substances like Omega 3 fats, you really can't get too much and every bit extra you do get will be of value.

ANTIOXIDANTS IN FOOD

Antioxidant	Source
lycopene, carotene	In citrus fruits (including marmalade because quantities are high in skin and pith), yellow and orange fruits and vegetables, apples, tea, tomatoes and all tomato products, and watermelon.
lutein, zeaxanthin	In kale, spinach and similar leafy green vegies, sweet corn, yellow and orange vegetables and fruit, egg yolks, pink-fleshed fish and seafood (including salmon and prawns).

flavonoids	In darker green vegetables like kale and spinach, broccoli, parsley, cauliflower, black teas, coffee (but not instant coffee), seaweed and all sorts of soy foods, apples, and citrus fruits.
anthocyanins	In red and purple fruits and vegetables including berries, red grapes and red wine, plums, eggplant skin, cherries, red lettuce or other vegetables with red or purple colour, raw cocoa powder and dark chocolate.
catechins	In apples, cocoa, white and green tea.
curcumin (turmeric spice)	This is the dark yellow spice used commonly in many Indian, Asian and middle eastern dishes.
other polyphenols	In coffee, green and black tea, whole grains, onions, garlic, ginger, mushrooms, flax seed, sesame seeds, lentils.
uridine	In tomatoes, brewer's yeast, broccoli, liver, molasses, and nuts.
choline	In egg yolk, meats and fish, whole grains.
Resveratrol	In peanuts, pistachios, red grape skins and red wine, blueberries, cocoa, dark chocolate
vitamin A	In all yellow and orange vegetables and fruits, as well as in eggs, butter, milk, cheese, and liver.
vitamin C	In citrus fruits, berries, mango, capsicums, potatoes, cabbage, spinach, and Asian greens.
vitamin E	In wheat germ (in wholemeal and wholegrain bread and cereals), vegetable oils, nuts, eggs, seeds, fish, and avocado.
selenium	In nuts (especially Brazil nuts) fish, seafood, liver, kidney, red meat, chicken, eggs, mushrooms, and grains. (The level of selenium in foods usually depends on how much is in the soil in which the food is grown.)
zinc	In lean red meat, liver, kidney, chicken, seafood (especially oysters), milk, whole grains, legumes, and nuts.
Carnosine	In the muscle of animals – higher in muscles that do a lot of exercise, so grass fed and wild meats will have more. Meats, chicken, fish, venison, rabbit, and any game meat.

Protection and function with water and fluids

Your brain cannot fire on all cylinders when you are even a little bit dehydrated no matter what your age. And if dehydration worsens it can present the brain with almost insurmountable challenges, bringing on confusion and incoherence surprisingly quickly, and with that getting more likely as you get older.

Without adequate hydration neurones just can't communicate with each other, which after all is what cognition is all about. Dehydration also affects blood flow through the brain, which results in a release of stress hormones. Excessive levels of these affect production of neurotransmitters and mess up the actions of not only the neurones themselves but also the glial cells so they can't supply the support and protection the neurones need.

As well, if you become unwell, even mild dehydration makes delirium far more likely – and that is a significant issue in itself for your brain as discussed in Chapter 1.

But even when you know all this, good hydration is often a challenge because increasing age means you don't feel thirsty as soon as you should. That happens for a whole lot of reasons summarised in the box here, but basically because some of the mechanisms that would usually be monitoring hydration levels and sending you messages to drink extra if they start to fall are affected by ageing – the messages just don't get though. So feeling thirsty becomes a less and less useful measure of fluid needs as you move into your later years. As well, some of those messages about thirst are combined with those about hunger, so if appetite declines for food, with it can go the messages to drink what the body needs. Appetite, how it changes, and what you can do about it are covered in detail in *Eat To Cheat Ageing*, if you need some assistance there.

SOME FACTORS CONTRIBUTING TO INCREASED CHANCE OF DEHYDRATION IN OLDER PEOPLE

Changes in the kidney's ability to retain water due to:

> altered hormone levels

> age-related loss of kidney function

Decreased sense of thirst

Diarrhoea or frequent loose motions (often resulting in reduced food/liquid intake)

Urinary incontinence and subsequent avoidance of drinking to reduce chance of accident.

Cognitive Impairment and Dementia

Fever

Heat stress

Blood loss due to injury or surgery

Medications – especially those with side effects that reduce thirst or appetite and of course diuretics that are designed to remove fluid from the body (the latter usually prescribed for heart conditions)

But suffice to say, when your food intake is down, so is the amount of fluid available to body and brain. That's partly because a lot of the water our bodies get each day comes from the food we eat. Also, we get some from the digestive process as foods are broken down. Therefore, not eating well makes dehydration even more likely.

MEDICATIONS THAT CAN PLAY A PART IN HYDRATION/DEHYDRATION

Diuretics (commonly called fluid tablets) are designed to remove excess fluid from your body, thus relieving some of the symptoms of heart problems. Keeping a balance between too much fluid affecting your heart and having enough to keep the rest of your body functioning is something that needs close monitoring by your doctor. It's essential to be aware that the dosage of these medications required can vary with weight loss and changes in your health so don't assume you always need to stay on the same dose of diuretic medication. And if you are unwell – especially with a fever – or heading for surgery adjustments may need to be made until you have recovered to avoid delirium and dehydration.

The brand names of diuretics include: *Lasix, Frusemide*

Other Medications that can contribute to dehydration

Laxatives – too numerous to specify brands

Angiotensin-converting enzyme inhibitors – brand names include:

Steroids

Psychotropics

Antipsychotics

Antidepressants

We do hold some fluid 'reserves' in our bodies that can provide temporary backup: but that's held largely in body muscle. Anyone who has lost weight and therefore muscle since their late 60s has also reduced that reserve so needs to be extra vigilant.

~ ~ ~

Water, Juice, Tea or Milk ?? – What and how much to drink to ward off dehydration

Most people should have between six to eight glasses or cups of liquid each day. Actually what you need is about 30ml of water for every kilogram you weigh (or 1 oz for every 2 pounds bodyweight) so you can work it out if you really want to. But that doesn't all have to come from water. In fact, for anyone that finds eating three good meals as well as the occasional snack a challenge each day, being pushed to drink lots of water can make things worse because filling up on water can mean not feeling like eating and missing out on valuable nutrients.

You get the fluid you need from many different sources: all sorts of drinks – including tea, coffee, juices, milk – and many different foods including fruits, soup, desserts, jelly, casseroles – anything not dry really.

For those who are eating well, ideally you will get what you need from water because you will be able to get in the food you need as well as extra water to fend off dehydration. Also, as long as you haven't unintentionally lost weight and are managing to eat well, then you won't need the extra energy (kilojoules or calories) that juices, soft drinks, milk etc. supply. Water is the best option.

But, if you have lost some weight or are struggling to eat well, then it's a very good idea to choose those extra energy drinks such as flavoured milk, protein shakes, and smoothies to boost your energy and nutrient-intake along with your fluids.

For most people a drink with each meal as well as something in between should give you enough fluids. Just be careful if you like to drink tea with your meals because it can affect how well you absorb some nutrients from the food in those meals. If you are not eating well then getting enough of some nutrients (especially iron) from food can be a challenge anyway so if possible, it's best to enjoy tea between meals.

If you are really struggling to eat, don't fill up on water before a meal if it's going to mean you won't feel like eating the food you need.

~ ~ ~

Fuelling the Brain

I said in *Eat To Cheat Ageing* that glucose is your brain's preferred fuel and that remains the case. Remember that even though it is only about two percent of your body weight, the brain is so metabolically active (a medical term for being really 'busy') it uses up a whopping 20 percent or more of your body's total energy supply. Keeping up with that sort of demand requires a dedicated fuel supply system, and that's always been understood to mean constant access to the blood sugar, glucose.

But the fabulous thing about medical research is that it's always peeling back layers to reveal more and more about the way our bodies work. That's been more challenging when it comes to the brain because of the excellent defences I've already mentioned. Work in the last decade when we have had the technology to allow us safe passage past those defences has revealed some useful things about fuelling the brain (some in only the couple of years since the research for *Eat To Cheat Ageing* was completed).

As mentioned above, the parts of the brain that keep all our 'background' body systems running – things like breathing, digesting, and keeping the heart beating and body organs functioning – use a pretty constant amount of fuel. When the areas involved in cognition come into play – the thinking processes of the brain, planning, analysing, observing, and making sense of things – that ramps up massively the amount of fuel needed, depending on what you are doing at the time. At these times, the demand for fuel is extremely high so even minor hiccups in supply are going to reduce cognitive ability.

~ ~ ~

Making the most of glucose

Research has shown that glucose use is lower in the brains of people who have dementia than in those that don't. But more than that, even before there are signs of cognitive decline, it looks like that might also be the case well before diagnosis. So reduced glucose use by the brain is a probable contributor to cognitive decline and dementia.

It's likely that it's not as much whether there is glucose available in the blood at any one time that is significant, but the ability of brain cells to get hold of and use it effectively that makes the difference between peak brain activity and anything below that.

Glucose needs to be able to get into brain cells to be used and that's quite a complex process. It involves the hormone insulin along with the combined actions of specialised 'carriers' to get it across the blood brain barrier. The important role of the glia in producing chemicals to cause a boost in blood flow to those especially active areas of the brain is vital. The extra blood flow gets more glucose and other resources to where they are needed and moves the additional waste produced by extra activity away from the neurones to protect them.

If any of these doesn't work as well as they should - if cells are resistant to the hormone insulin (as happens in type 2 diabetes and in insulin resistance or pre-diabetes), if any or all of the glucose carriers don't do their job, or if the blood vessels don't open adequately - that limits the brain's ability to access and use glucose and results in an overall lower glucose use..

One or all of these are certainly part of the picture in dementia:

It's at times when the demand is especially high that insulin would usually give an extra glucose boost so insulin resistance is a particular problem for the brain, reducing its ability to get the glucose it needs when it needs it most. You will read more on the part played by insulin resistance and the condition now often called Type 3 diabetes linked to dementia in Chapter 6.

A quick note though before we move on, on the part played by omega 3 fats in fuelling the brain. They can't be used as fuel themselves but the omega 3 fat known as DHA helps the neurones access and use glucose as well as assisting the brain in many other ways. The brains of people with Alzheimer's disease have lower levels of DHA and use less glucose than those without Alzheimer's, so it's very likely they are linked but it's not exactly clear how yet.

The other two omega 3 fats also seem to be important: ALA and EPA are both involved in bolstering either fuel supply to cells by supporting glucose availability, or by boosting ketone supply (read on for more on this) for times when glucose just isn't in adequate supply. ALA can also be converted to DHA to increase its availability.

As I said, we know that the areas of the brain affected in people with Alzheimer's disease are routinely using less glucose (and therefore achieving less) than those of people without Alzheimer's and it was widely assumed that was a 'result' of damage caused by that disease. But it could well in fact be the reverse: many now believe that a reduced ability to fuel brain cells is actually one of the 'causes' of brain changes that eventually manifest as Alzheimer's and possibly other dementias.

Not only are under-fuelled cells unable to do what you need of them day to day, but they also become more susceptible to oxidative stress, inflammation, and the build-up of substances like β amyloid.

THE VITAL IMPORTANCE TO YOUR BRAIN OF MERELY EATING

It may seem improbable but the day will likely arrive when your appetite will not constantly persuade you to make the most of every morsel that comes your way. Appetite makes mistakes – if it didn't, everyone on the planet would be the ideal weight all their lives without needing to access the dreaded 'will power' at all, and this is certainly not the case. Allowing your appetite to convince you that you don't need to eat so much now you are older, that it's OK to skip meals, or that a few mouthfuls make up an adequate meal, put your brain at risk.

Of course, you might not think about eating if you are busy with other things or you might believe that because you're not doing as much you don't need as much as you used to. Nothing could be further from the truth: at the very least, your nutrient needs are the same as they have been all your adult life –some things you actually need more of. To make the most of the years you have as well as counter the effects of ageing on the brain, eating well so you get the fuel and nutrients your brain needs is even more important now.

What's more, the mere routine of eating three or more meals a day plays a vital role because eating is a habit thing. You can just as easily get in the habit of missing meals as you once may have been in the habit of a little extra ice cream on your desert, and that can be the start of a slippery slope into malnutrition, which clearly will not help your brain.

I covered issues with appetite in *Eat To Cheat Ageing* and if yours has decreased at all, have a look there, where problems with appetite and how to deal with them are covered in more detail.

~ ~ ~

Getting a fuel boost – the role of ketones in the brain in Alzheimer's and other dementias

The brain will always need glucose in its fuel mix, but it is able to employ some strategies to access backup fuel when glucose supply is inadequate: it can use substances called ketones. However, managing to supply these to the cells where they are needed is not without challenges.

You don't get ketones from food and they are not as simple to make as glucose. We have always known ketones were made by the liver from body fat or fat in food after that had been broken down into fatty acids (fat's smallest components), but till now we believed that mostly only happened when a person was starving (and I mean really starving, not just complaining loudly of hunger!).

During starvation (or in extended fasts or extreme 'ketogenic' diets designed to mimic starvation) the brain puts the pressure on for fuel and its needs are very high compared to other body systems. It quickly uses up the limited glucose supplies and muscle protein is converted into glucose to add to those, but with no food coming in at all, that still isn't always enough. The cells in the rest of the body can use body fat in the form of fatty acids to bolster their energy supplies, but the brain can't use fatty acids as fuel, starvation or not. The liver swings into action, converting fatty acids into ketones and they *can* be used by fuel hungry brain cells.

This is great because the brain can work well with ketones as a supplementary fuel. BUT (yes, there is often a 'but') those brain cells that for whatever reason are under-using glucose and might benefit from a regular supply of ketones to help out are not going to get them unless you are 'actually' starving because the liver doesn't normally make them. So there has been a lot of interest in the past few years in manipulating the diet to get the liver making more ketones to possibly boost brain capacity when it's not using glucose as well as it should.

Diets that 'push' the liver to make ketones are called 'ketogenic' and are not new. In the past, they've been used in two main ways. They have been used in weight loss because they encourage the use of body fat, but they are pretty extreme and most people find them challenging because they contain no carbohydrate foods – no bread, cereals, rice, grains or foods made from them, no milk, no fruit, no sugar, and restrictions on many vegetables – and are high in fat. Not only that, but they rarely achieve long-term success as the resumption of a more usual diet mostly results in weight regain.

However, they have also been used to treat severe epilepsy in children and it is from this use, recognising they can have effects on brain function that they come into our discussion here.

The logic says that if the brains of those with cognitive decline and dementia might benefit from an extra supply of ketones and that ketogenic diets can help in a brain condition like epilepsy, maybe they can help in cognitive decline and dementia too. So it was with great anticipation that researchers started to look at using these diets to boost cognition in people with cognitive decline and dementia. But the findings haven't been as good as was hoped and these strict ketogenic diets are not easy for anyone, let alone someone living with dementia who would find them too unusual and challenging to manage most of the time.

So more recently that strict ketogenic diet has been modified using a type of fat called medium chain triglyceride (MCT). This is an interesting type of fat because it's able to bypass that conversion into fatty acids that other fats have to go through before they can be made into ketones in the liver. Because MCTs can be converted directly into ketones it was thought that might be a big plus when brain glucose use was down. This newer modified ketogenic diet doesn't require the severe restriction of carbohydrate foods that the older ones did so is easier to manage. In addition, there has been some evidence that this does help some people, but unfortunately, that is not as universal as was hoped.

The most abundant source of MCTs in food is coconut or coconut oil, which is now widely marketed in organic, virgin and all manner of other forms but that I knew as copha from my blissful childhood chocolate crackle making days! MCTs are now also supplied in commercial MCT oil preparations. Manufacturers of these oils and coconut products have widely promoted the benefits of the MCT diet in treating dementia, even claiming preventive abilities, but unfortunately again the science is not always as encouraging as the marketing claims. Read more in the text box here.

~ ~ ~

SOME THOUGHTS ON COCONUT OIL AND MCTS

I'm not a fan of most widely promoted 'new' diets but I'm also a realist. If there is a strategy that seems to do no harm but might help some people then it may be worth a try, so here is my take on this idea and a few things to watch out for.

The proponents of coconut oil and other MCT diets suggest working up to at least 3 tablespoons per day to achieve benefits. There are a couple of things to be aware of if you are even thinking of this:

- Coconut oil is the most saturated fat in our diet, but a high proportion of the fats it contains are 'medium chain triglycerides' (MCTs) which are a type of saturated fat and thus it is naturally a solid at shelf temperature like other saturated fats (think butter, lamb or beef fat and most coconut oil). You will know its a genuine, unchanged coconut oil product if it is solid at room or shelf temperature - but that can make it challenging to use (it needs to be heated or melted to be incorporated into most foods or cooked into things and can't easily be added to cold foods or drinks). Nowadays you can buy coconut oil that is liquid but be aware it is not the same product.

- One of the MCTs coconut oil contains (lauric acid) is more solid at shelf temperature than the rest. Removing that by processing results in a liquid that can still be called coconut oil despite its different composition. The reason lauric acid is removed is not for any therapeutic benefit but because it has a number of commercial uses in other food products and beyond: it's also used in an amazing array of non-food things ranging from soaps and cosmetics to medications and cleaning products.

- Lauric acid is also found in abundance in human breast milk so is important for the developing brain of a baby and probably, in an adult brain along with other MCTs.
Don't believe that liquid coconut oil is the same as solid - it is not.

- Commercial MCT oils (not labelled coconut oil) are not naturally occurring products but result from commercial blending of selected MCTs to produce a specific therapeutic liquid product that can be added to cold foods and drinks.

- Diets high in coconut oil may cause diarrhoea so if you are going to try one, start with just a teaspoon and work up if there are no ill effects.

- Because diets high in coconut oil can be somewhat unpalatable, it can be sometimes be challenging to get foods accepted. Try adding the oil to cooked or hot foods where possible and including the flesh of the coconut for its fibre is a good idea.

- Unfortunately, the internet tends to loudly proclaim the benefits some individuals have found from all sorts of diets that claimed to have changed lives. In contrast, disappointing results naturally are unlikely to be shared widely. MCT and coconut oil diet strategies have worked for some and there have been some larger scale studies recently that have found benefits. But it's hard to separate the benefits that the high MCT and therefore high kJ (calorie) intake may have provided in terms of helping avoid malnutrition from those of the MCTs themselves. I think until the science is clear on this, my best advice is that it's worth a try and it is unlikely to do harm as long as you take it slowly.

- It's always best when it has had to undergo processing to choose coconut oil that has undergone minimal extraction processing so not only may it not be worth the effort unless you can be assured a reputable supply but the good stuff can be very costly to buy the best product. There are plenty of recipes on the internet you can try.

- Companies promoting their own coconut oil or MCT products are always keen to increase their market so beware of claims made – they may not necessarily be wrong or excessive but it's important to always check who is making them and what their motivation might be.

- There are many outspoken supporters of ketogenic diets and especially coconut oil diets and for some people they may help at least for a time, buying valuable time. But there is no good evidence that they have useful long-term benefits in those already experiencing cognitive decline. It could be that people start on ketogenic diets when β amyloid build-up and other dementia contributors are already well advanced. But if they do work for an individual, they may improve cognitive abilities for a time.

Recently advanced technology in neuroscience has produced a big revelation about ketones: the astrocytes (a type of glia) in the brain are able to make ketones themselves. Astrocytes assist neurones in many ways and providing a supply of ketones might just be one of those with the power to help maintain brain health. It's when astrocytes are affected by inflammation and oxidative stress that they might lose some or all of that ability.

There is a long way to go in our understanding of this whole area. But certainly doing all that is possible to help the astrocytes out certainly can't do any harm – and that's the same as supporting every other cell in the body – reducing oxidative stress and chronic inflammation that it covered ad nauseum in this book and *Eat To Cheat Ageing*.

Of course, in more frail individuals and in people living with dementia, eating very small quantities of food that may induce a type of starvation state is quite common. The brains of these individuals probably rely on ketones quite often, but the other effects of reduced food intake on muscle and the rest of the body probably outweigh any benefits that provides.

~ ~ ~

SUGAR IS SUGAR IS SUGAR IS SUGAR – RIGHT?

Don't get the blood sugar glucose mixed up with sugars from food. When the media and the popular press mention sugar, what they mean usually is sucrose, or sugars like fructose from fruit, HFCS (high fructose corn syrup), agave syrup, honey or other.

Sucrose is the sugar derived from sugar cane. HFCS is an industrial product derived from maize (corn) that is cheaper and a bit sweeter than cane sugar so is often used in manufactured foods and drinks. Agave juice is a bit of a recent fad in western countries – being derived from the sap of a South American plant. Honey we all know and love…all are types of sugar.

Blood glucose is completely different – certainly it's derived or can be derived from sucrose or any of the sugars above, but also from any other carbohydrate in the diet including rice, pasta , bread, and fruit - it is the preferred fuel for every cell in the body to achieve what it needs to do every second. The level of glucose in the blood is regulated by the hormone insulin and there is a lot more on the role of insulin and the contribution that insulin resistance and type-2 diabetes make to dementia in Chapter 6.

Chapter 3

GETTING THE FOUNDATIONS RIGHT – PREPARE YOUR BODY TO SUPPORT YOUR BRAIN

Thomas Edison said, "The chief function of the body is to carry the brain around."

That might be a bit of an oversimplification but he does have a point. Unless you support your body, it is not going to be able to carry your brain around. Moreover, since your muscles also help protect vulnerable brain cells from the damage done by inflammation, it's essential we review what they need.

Eat To Cheat Ageing covered the body beyond the muscles if you need a wider discussion.

Muscle is what we are looking at here because it does so much more than most people are aware. Your muscles are made of protein and they do more than help you move around, they contribute a vital reserve supply of protein and its component amino acids, to be used day in and day out for a wide variety of body functions including fuelling the brain.

Protein is needed to maintain every one of your body's organs: every cell in each one — in your skin, your gut, your blood cells, bone tissue, liver, heart, kidneys and every other body organ — has a lifespan. Constant renewal is always underway: some cells have only hours of life, some days, some months before they are replaced with new ones and it's protein that is demanded minute by minute for this vital task.

Protein also provides so many of the substances that keep systems running – enzymes for digestion, hormones to instruct body systems, neurotransmitters to allow the brain to function. It's essential to fight illness and infection by supplying immune substances.

Then there is repair work that ranges from healing everyday cuts and bruises to accidents that are more significant, and injuries, right through to the mammoth reconstruction work needed on muscle, surrounding tissue, bone, and tendon after major surgery.

Last but certainly not least, that same muscle protein supplies neurotransmitters and back-up fuel to your brain so it also underpins cognitive processes.

But protein comes from food surely, so why the need to use muscles as a supply depot?

As I explained in *Eat To Cheat Ageing*, It's rather like your car. Once you turn that key, you expect to be able to travel many miles or kilometres. Your car needs fuel to keep running but you don't carry the petrol station (or the power point if you have entered the brave new world of electric cars) around with you for that constant supply. Your car's fuel tank is your reserve between fill ups. Muscle is our protein reserve between food fill ups. But unlike our cars, which we can switch off when the day's work is done, there is always a need for protein somewhere in your body, day and night — even when you are sleeping — so the protein fuel tank (your muscles), is always in use.

Protein is released from your muscles to bridge any gaps between food fill ups. Those gaps come along surprisingly often: there are many non-eating hours between meals; there are times when you struggle to eat at all if you are unwell; and there are times you actively avoid food for medical, religious, or other reasons, not to mention those days when, somehow, you just don't get time to eat the meals you should.

For most of life, we have more than enough muscle to do all the tasks our body needs to do and any moved out is quickly replaced when we next eat. But a combination of changes in the efficiency of replacing muscle protein as you move into your later years with the adding up of lots and lots of small losses over the years results in a gradual decline in muscle reserve. That can eventually mean that immunity, organ maintenance, and all the backup roles that protein reserve usually assists with including providing fuel and resources to the brain, just won't work, as they should. I often think if we only lived till early 70s – and let's face it, it wasn't long ago that that was as long as we were expected to live – the muscle reserves built as we grew into adulthood would hold out. But with decades to enjoy beyond 70 nowadays we need them not only to hold out but to help us get the most out of the time ahead.

The take away message is that you must do all you can to support your muscles so they can continue to keep you active as well as assist your body and brain. Because make no mistake, allowing that protein reserve to dwindle will hamper both body and brain function.

Supporting muscles requires combining muscle activity with eating protein foods – more on that later. First, a bit of background on why age doesn't help our muscles very much and what you can do about it.

MUSCLE IS NEEDED TO:

stop you from falling if you should lose balance or miss your step

allow you to keep exercising effectively and moving around safely

support your joints to reduce the pain of arthritis and similar conditions and maintain your flexibility

support the function of your heart, lungs and every other body organ

help you to continue to swallow safely and effectively

help boost your appetite

help your body use insulin effectively to avoid diabetes developing or worsening

keep fuel supplied to your brain

help you avoid having an adverse reaction to a medication

~ ~ ~

Balancing losses with rebuilding – age strikes again

It's usual for protein to move in and out of muscles in response to supply and demand. Bodies growing into healthy adulthood are hard-wired to build muscle. And if any was lost while your muscle reserve was temporarily doing its rescue work, you were conveniently programmed to rebuild it as soon as you ate again.

But that programmed rebuilding requires a combination of three things:

> messages from hormones
>
> signals from nerves
>
> the activity of muscles themselves.

Here's where our bodies' ageist physiology strikes. Hormone levels diminish and the signals from nerves dwindle with age. From as early as your 30s or 40s, both are affected and, by your mid 60s, hormone and nerve boosting of muscle has all but ceased.

That leaves muscle activity alone in the rebuilding task. But, your muscles are reminded to repair and build only when you work them. Fortunately, even though it gets more difficult to rebuild the older you get, that system does keep working into your later years.

So if your body is to have any chance at all of keeping pace with the plans you've made for the years ahead, it needs your help.

Those flabby arms and bingo wings, flibberty bits, saggy bottoms, and turkey necks might be gravity's joke but under that exterior, it's up to you to nurture your inner Adonis.

That means considering five things:

Ironically, after all those years when most of us seemed to struggle to keep our meal sizes within civilized boundaries, when we were often being told to eat less meat and dairy and that the pinnacle of good nutrition was a plate piled to the ceiling with salad and veggies topped with nothing but a squeeze of lemon, the time has now come when a lot of that will get turned on its head. Not everyone is going to find themselves eating less and less food as they get older, but improbable as it seems, very many of us will. In addition, while all those lovely vegetables, fruits, and leafy things provide irreplaceable vitamin and antioxidant boosters, the meats and cheeses of this world take on an elevated status from now on.

Why? Because you are still running an adult-sized body, no matter how old you are and it still has adult-sized needs for most nutrients. In fact, with all the extra wear and tear amassed as the years pile up, you need more of some things than you did when you were younger — and protein is one — so the importance of packing extra nutrition into your meals to keep your muscles up to scratch and cheat ageing is undeniable. You don't have to eat huge amounts of those protein foods but you mustn't eat less than you did when younger.

Too often protein foods get forgotten on the plate, becoming more of a garnish than a focus in a meal or somehow thought of as dispensable. But nothing could be further from the truth: because protein needs are in fact a bit higher, not lower, as you age many will need to look at ways to get a bit more, not less.

GOOD SOURCES OF PROTEIN

All meats, fish, poultry and seafood	all fresh cuts or processed — including ham, bacon, smoked meat, poultry and sausages, and all products containing red meats, poultry, and fish.
Dairy foods	including milk, cheese, yoghurt (but excluding cream and butter) also milks, cheeses and yoghurt from goats and sheep

Soy products	including soy milk, yoghurt, tofu, tempeh, and others
Pulses	including lentils, chick peas, dried beans, and peas
All nuts and seeds	and products made from them
Whole grains	and products made from them

~ ~ ~

But life is too short to spend on having to think about every mouthful you take. So make it easy on yourself.

Just put a protein food at the centre of most meals from now on and you won't have to struggle to get what you need.

When you ate larger meals, you could easily get away with having protein foods only at some meals or in very small amounts as a 'garnish' while vegetables, fruits, and grains held centre stage. In fact that's the ideal diet plan to combat obesity in younger people and is, what you will often hear or read is right for older as well as younger adults. However, unless you include a good protein food at most meals you risk not being able to cope with your body's demand. And, don't forget, if you do suffer an illness or an infection you will need to eat even more protein to help balance what your muscles will lose. That means eating protein between meals and, for many, adding high protein drinks or supplements.

2. Animal vs vegetable protein

Let's face it, if you need more protein than years ago but don't want to eat bigger meals or if you are finding yourself eating less than you once did, then it stands to reason you need to pack more protein and other essentials into every serving.

That means animal foods have the advantage because your servings of meat, fish, egg or dairy food don't need to be as large to get the same amount of protein as they do when it comes from most plant foods (such as soy milk, nuts, seeds and grains).

We also know from sports science that animal protein is able to help build muscles in athletes more than most plant proteins can, especially if it's eaten close to the time when you exercise (ideally within an hour). Building and maintaining muscle is of course of immense importance to athletes, but even if you are not planning to run a four-minute mile any day soon, your muscles will still benefit in the same way and the stakes are higher: building and maintaining muscle provides the key to body and brain health from now on.

Years ago, concerns about fat and cholesterol may have had you cutting down on meat, eggs, and dairy but those concerns don't stack up the same way as you advance in age. Protein is now so very important and the other nutrients those foods supply are a decided bonus. It's not about eating only protein foods, or eating large amounts but getting quality protein foods at every meal. Low fat diets are no longer what is most needed. It's time to ditch those concerns that may well have been quite right for us as young adults – time to enjoy one of the benefits of reaching a more mature age!

While it's always best to get protein from meals so you also get the benefit of the nutrients in the accompanying foods, occasionally you might need to add high protein drinks (there's a lot more on boosting protein including recipes for supplement drinks and eating plans in *Eat To Cheat Ageing*). The array of supplements in the supermarket aisles can be bewildering but those based on the dairy product, whey (whey protein isolate or whey protein concentrate), are considered to do the best job. If you are vegan or vegetarian, you might prefer formulas based on soy protein isolate.

You are not going to achieve a Charles Atlas body, or whoever his svelte female counterpart might be. However, supplements might just give you the boost your muscles need at times when you are not able to get a good serving of protein at each meal (and in between meals if you need the extra if you are ill or recovering from illness).

PROTEIN CONTENT IN FOODS AND THEIR EFFECTIVENESS IN PROMOTING MUSCLE GROWTH

Food type (listed in order of the general ability of the protein they contain to boost muscle growth)	The amount of food needed for 20 to 30g protein per meal (the ideal muscle boost quantity) (listed for each food)
Whey protein isolate powder	20g (approx. 1 dessertspoon)
Meat or fish (cooked)	100g (size of a regular pack of cards or 1 small tin of tuna or salmon)
Skim milk powder	60g powder (approx. 2 tablespoons or 600ml liquid skim milk)
Egg	3 eggs
Milk	600ml (or approx. 80g or 3 dessertspoons milk powder)
Cottage cheese	140g
Cheese (cheddar or similar)	3 slices of processed cheese or equivalent sized amount
Yoghurt	400g (large tub)
Soy protein isolate powder	20g (approx. 1 dessertspoon)
Soy milk	900ml
Lentils	400g can
Almonds	about 95 nuts or 130g (1 cup)
Tofu	200g (about the size of 2 packs of cards)
Rice (cooked)	6 cups
Bread (sliced)	9 slices

~ ~ ~

Like you and me, muscles like to be reminded they're needed. There's no getting round the saying, 'use it or lose it'. Sure, it's harder to keep your muscles the way they were, but unless you keep using them, and using them well, they'll forget what they're there for.

That means you need to think about the type of muscle activity you do. First, there's the benefit of gravity. Our muscles thrive on the effects of gravity and you can use that to your advantage by avoiding sitting or lying down too much. Of course you need to rest but don't get complacent, keep looking for ways that gravity can help you every day: get up, stand tall, move around, carry things, use the stairs, park further from the shop, walk instead of drive, rake the lawn, sweep the floor. There are endless examples.

And then there is exercise itself. Sadly, it's just not enough anymore to stroll around the shops or to go for a leisurely walk. In order to boost muscle function at every chance, you need to do activities that stress your muscles and help make up for those absent hormones and vastly diminished nerve triggers.

Because you have muscles everywhere, it has to be activity that works not only your legs, but also your upper body, arms and abdomen. Your muscles need to work against a weight (called resistance exercise) to encourage them to build. Luckily, 'resistance' doesn't only mean lifting weights in a gym. Aquarobic exercise or swimming laps uses the water as resistance. Walking briskly or uphill, sweeping, or raking the leaves instead of waving the leaf blower about, taking the stairs more often, even doing supervised exercises like tai chi or 'over 50's' fitness classes, are all good as long as they get your heart rate up and have you puffing and sweating a little. (There is a list of suggested activities to maintain your muscles below.)

All these activities need to be checked with your doctor first of course and carefully supervised as you get older, but that doesn't mean you shouldn't do them. Accepting age as a reason to do less and less physical activity, to sit most of the day and to have lots of daytime naps, as too many do, will only do you harm in the long run.

As soon as you are able after an illness or after being immobilised for any time, you will need to work extra hard to help recover what you might have lost. It may not be what you feel like doing, but it will certainly help you out when you are faced with any similar challenges. (See the extra suggestions for recovery below.)

The rules about what is good for you now that you are older are not the same as those that applied when you were younger. If you could count on living only until your late 60s, your muscle reserves may well hold out without much help. But as you are likely to live well past those years, your health and independence in the future depends on those reserves still being there when you need them in your 80s and beyond. And that won't happen without you making an effort.

GUIDELINES FOR EXERCISE TO HELP MAINTAIN MUSCLE FUNCTION

The ideal is to combine aerobic, resistance, flexibility, and balance activities, so you need to find activities, which you are able to do, which don't put you at risk of falling and ideally, which interest you. Professional assistance is ideal but not essential. Everyday activities like vacuuming, mopping, raking, sweeping, gardening, carrying the shopping, and doing housework also contribute but adopting the following are your best bet to cheat ageing:

Aerobic

on at least 3 days per week initially, increasing to every day

aim for 30 to 60 minutes each day, which can be accumulated in 10 minute bouts

make at least 20 or 30 minutes of this time at vigorous intensity (puffing and sweating)

Resistance

weight training on at least 2 days per week

exercises for all major muscle groups: legs, arms, abdomen, hips, back, chest, shoulders

repeat each exercise 8 to 12 times

increase the weight you lift as it gets easier or repeat more times

Flexibility

sustained stretches for each major muscle group on at least 2 days per week

use static stretches, not those involving movement

Balance

on at least 1 day and eventually up to 7 days do 4 to 10 different balance activities in a safe environment only, repeat each 1 or 2 times

There is more detailed information, in the appendix of this book, including exercises and how to measure your exercise intensity.

EXERCISE GUIDELINES
FOR RECOVERY AFTER ILLNESS OR IMMOBILISATION

Resistance exercise is the most important for recovery. Don't expect it to increase the size of your muscles as that's unlikely, but it will help in your recovery, boost your strength and ability, and improve your longer-term health.

You can start with either no weights, or very light ones, but add extra when you can, or do extra repetitions on the same weight so you progress in strength.

As soon as you are able — even while you are confined to bed (and as long as it's safe to do so) — start to do as much as you can even if it's only one or two activities at first.

Work up to doing 8 to 12 repetitions of exercises for each major muscle group: legs, arms, abdomen, hips, back, chest, and shoulders.

If you have had surgery or an injury and are in the hospital, check what you are able to do with the physiotherapist or ask your doctor.

As soon as you are able, return to doing all your maintenance activities.

~ ~ ~

Being immobilised through illness — also somewhat misleadingly called 'bed rest' — is more harmful to your muscles than merely leading an inactive life. It affects your body in much the same way as being in zero gravity for an astronaut, and the more so the older you get. Lying around robs you of muscle and once you are older it doesn't come back automatically.

If you have had an accident, surgery or sickness, chances are you will spend some time in bed and during that time your muscles won't get their usual workout. In addition, that workout includes the everyday fight against gravity to keep you upright as well as everything else you do to remind your muscles what they are there for. So, although you may not feel like doing anything more active than eating delightful hospital cuisine and drinking stewed tea while you are confined to bed, you are going to lose muscle if you don't get up as soon as you can, or at least do some exercise while you are there.

There is a silver lining: some of the lost muscle becomes protein reserve and is diverted into repairing wounds, combating infection, or fighting off fever.

Unfortunately, the combined losses through diversion into repair work and the lack of exercise can be very large. Realising what's going on and working to minimise the effects can be your key to stopping a vicious cycle of muscle loss and illness, which then could potentially trigger increasing frailty and chronic ill health. Get active as soon as you are able, so that muscle loss won't become permanent.

Be clear, you might also lose body fat with any of this type of weight loss, but that's not the bonus you might think it is because weight loss during immobilisation, illness, or after surgery is a sign all-important muscle has certainly also been lost.

If the time in bed is only a day or two, there's little to be worried about, enjoy the rest. However, over a period of 10 days or so, it can easily rob you of 1kg of body muscle — a lot to lose. (See below for a perspective on muscle loss.)

Daytime rests can also be an issue if they get out of hand. A nanna nap can certainly be replenishing, but too much rest time every day just means your muscles are missing out.

HOW MUCH MUSCLE DO I HAVE AND HOW CAN LOSING IT AFFECT ME?

The amount of muscle we have varies enormously depending on how much resistance exercise we do regularly. For most moderately active people in the healthy weight range muscle is usually about 40 percent of bodyweight.

Muscle loss increases your chance of gaining excess weight and your likelihood of developing type 2 diabetes, or hampering management if you already have diabetes.

During a major illness, losing just five percent of body muscle reduces the function of your internal organs and slows wound healing.

With a loss of around 20 percent of body muscle, organs begin to fail.

Death can result from a 40 percent loss of body muscle.

For an older person weighing between 65 and 70kg, you could easily lose five percent of your body muscle by losing 5kg of bodyweight.

~ ~ ~

5. The problem of an over-enthusiastic immune system

Your immune system is able to rally the 'protein troops' to mount a defence almost the instant a foreign substance enters the body. It's working before you're even aware you've been invaded, and it can neutralise a threat before any symptoms get the chance to appear.

It's an awesome response plan and it efficiently protects you from illness. Your muscle releases protein to be converted into specialised immune substances as soon as the system starts up and keeps doing so as long as it's active. But, as you age, the system can become overactive so that your muscles release protein to the immune system more often, or for longer than they should. Small amounts of muscle can continue to be lost even when you have recovered or are feeling quite well — often over quite long periods of time. Sometimes your immune system can also react when there is no real threat and that's a big problem for your muscles because targeting unwanted invaders uses muscle protein.

You won't always know it's happening, though weight loss might be a tell-tale sign. Nevertheless, you should always assume that you actively need to rebuild your muscle reserves after any illness now that you are older.

The same recovery strategies you need to put in place after immobilisation will also help head off any lingering losses after illness.

It's easy and mostly common sense to avoid muscle loss setting you up for ill health, but so many people inadvertently make choices that don't help. Muscle can be lost for many years before stick-thin arms and legs make it physically obvious and, all the while, the body's systems, which rely on that muscle protein reserve, can be faltering. It's hard to reverse if it goes on too long: avoidance is so much easier.

All this talk of eating more seems to fly in the face of what you may read about eating plans, which restrict food intake, or encourage weight loss to boost health benefits. But these plans are not things you should suddenly take up if you are closer to 90 than 50. The big issues round weight control and ageing are covered in greater detail in *Eat To Cheat Ageing*, and elsewhere in this book.

Chapter 4

BRAIN NUTRIENTS

Your brain needs nutrients for many things. Fuel for all the things it needs to do was covered in the previous chapter – here we will look at the nutrients that help make the neurotransmitters that allow it to communicate between cells, and those that keep it healthy and protected.

~ ~ ~

It does seem that age reduces the activity of all neurotransmitters and we don't know why but it stands to reason that it will affect cognition.

~ ~ ~

Making neurotransmitters

Neurotransmitters work throughout the body in every neurone and in the digestive tract, facilitating communication between the gut bacteria. The gut bacteria make their own, but they are also influenced by those released on instruction from the brain into the gut. The brain has to make its own because neurotransmitters cannot cross the blood brain barrier, although there are substances produced by the gut bacteria that are able to cross and influence the brain's neurotransmitter production.

Different neurotransmitters are made from specific amino acids (building blocks of proteins) that need to be brought in across the blood brain barrier.

You have already heard how the blood brain barrier acts like a security cordon to protect the highly vulnerable brain from potential unwanted intruders. It's great at that job, but unfortunately, like any security barrier, it can slow down the passage of things you do want to get in as much as things you don't. And the extra step means the amount of each that can be made at any time, and how quickly, can be restricted.

Of course, the blood brain barrier allows nutrients through, but in the case of amino acids, it acts a bit like a car ferry on a river crossing: safe passage is assured but only so many vehicles can get across at any one time. There are specific 'ferries' for amino acids, but only a certain number of them and the ferry operators don't play favourites – it's a first-in-first-served system. So even though brain cells may be waiting on the other side for specific amino acids to make specific neurotransmitters, the ones they need have to wait in line with other amino acids being ferried over for different tasks – it's not hard to see how easily that can slow production down, especially at times when the needs are high.

There have been ideas put forward, and you may have even read advice about foods or supplements you can eat to boost certain brain chemicals (such as boosting serotonin by taking supplements or eating foods high in tryptophan to reduce depression). The idea is that, by providing the particular amino acids that are used in the manufacture of the neurotransmitter, you can get the brain to make extra of that one.

However, the blood brain barrier gets in the way of that, literally and figuratively, because we eat amino acids in proteins that contain all sorts of amino acids (most having no association at all with neurotransmitters) and it's only during digestion that the amino acids are released from those proteins. After that, they have to deal with the ferryman and when a meal has contained lots of different amino acids, there is no guarantee that the ones needed will make it across quickly.

In addition, as discussed in much greater detail in Chapter 7, the gut microbiome has been found to produce at least one neurotransmitter, GABA, and impact the production of others, particularly serotonin.

With serotonin, it seems the gut bacteria impact the brain's access to tryptophan, which is needed for its production. Maybe there is some bribery of the ferryman going on in getting certain substances across, but whatever the way it's happening, it may not be the blend of amino acids you are taking in a supplement as much as the way you support your gut bacteria that matters. The finer points of this system are certainly not clear yet, but even though taking supplements or eating certain foods to attempt to manipulate neurotransmitter production may seem like it will work, unfortunately, it doesn't always achieve that.

Some care has to be taken with attempts to manipulate brain chemistry of course. Eating foods reputed to be high in certain amino acids is very unlikely to do harm because nothing is made entirely of one type. But taking a supplement is more like taking medication and might do more harm than good if it's not done under medical supervision: just because something isn't made by a pharmaceutical company, doesn't mean it won't act like a medication with side effects and therapeutic implications.

~ ~ ~

And then there is the added issue that the same 'ferries' that transport amino acids sometimes also have to take things other than amino acids across, thus potentially slowing, or at least complicating things further. Incidentally that includes the Parkinson's Disease medication levodopa (brand names include *Madopar, Sinemet*) and is one of the reasons it can be extra difficult to effectively treat Parkinson's Disease symptoms as the medication has to compete with other amino acids from protein foods. Levodopa is a variety of the neurotransmitter dopamine.

~ ~ ~

Once the necessary amino acids do make it into the brain, they need to be manufactured into the appropriate neurotransmitter in processes that need a wide array of substances to help make that happen, all of which also have to make it through the security cordon. Vitamins, minerals, antioxidant substances, and certain fatty acids (including Omega 3 oils) are all needed for this work.

Many things influence the levels of various neurotransmitters including stress, alcohol, inadequate diet, neurotoxins, both recreational and therapeutic drugs, and exercise. Only exercise and a beneficial diet have positive effects – the rest over the years may lead to imbalances and reduced ability to supply what the brain needs in later life.

SOME NEUROTRANSMITTERS AND A POTTED LOOK AT WHAT THEY DO

It's worth mentioning firstly that we can measure levels of neurotransmitters in blood but at this stage can't do that in the working brain itself and because of the blood brain barrier, we just don't know whether the blood levels are related at all to those in the brain.

Serotonin

This is the one targeted by the most common antidepressants, the SSRIs (selective serotonin reuptake inhibitors) and related medications intended to boost levels if they fall too low. It's the one that, at the right level, gives people a positive outlook and reduces anxiety and stress levels. Depression is not dementia of course, but when depression occurs in later age, they do seem to be linked. Scientists looking at the brains of people who have passed away have found that there are lower levels of serotonin in the brains of people who had Alzheimer's compared to those that didn't, but just observing that doesn't give any answers because it's not clear if the Alzheimer's caused the reduced levels or the other way round. Because of that, it's not clear if increasing levels of serotonin will be able to treat or delay dementia, but interestingly a healthy gut microbiome, which is associated with better cognition, does tend to increase its levels in the brain.

Serotonin also has roles in memory, learning, sleep, and social behaviour and many more things of less relevance to dementia. In depression, it seems that either there is a reduction in the amount being made, or it's not recognised as it should be and thus can't achieve what it would usually be able to, or a combination of the two. It is made in the brain and the gut from the amino acid tryptophan.

GABA

This one supports the nervous system and plays a critical role in mental alertness, elevated mood, and avoiding depression, and imbalances are associated with aggressive behaviour. It is made from the amino acid glutamic acid and its production by gut bacteria affects brain levels.

Dopamine

The brain's reward and pleasure centres are largely controlled by dopamine along with its involvement in regulating movement and emotional responses. It's what has probably made us successful as humans because it regulates competitiveness and aggression. This neurotransmitter is impacted in Parkinson's disease where inadequate supply most obviously causes movement issues, but also can contribute in time to a type of dementia. In contrast, an oversupply (that happens when taking some illicit drugs, particularly methamphetamines) causes severe aggression and euphoria. It is made in the brain from the amino acid tyrosine.

Norepinephrine (or noradrenaline)

This is involved in heightening body and brain activity levels and awareness. It's also important in embedding memories, in other words holding onto things seen or experienced so they stick around for later. It is also manufactured from tyrosine in another step along from dopamine.

NUTRIENTS ESSENTIAL TO PEAK BRAIN FUNCTION

Glucose for brain fuel

Fatty acids and micro-nutrients for protection and function:

omega-3 fatty acids

The vitamins:

> Antioxidant vitamins A, C, and E

> B1, B3 (niacin), B6, B12, folate, and vitamin D

The minerals:

> Iodine, iron, magnesium, selenium and zinc

Maintenance and protection

Neurones are not continually renewed in quite the same way most body cells are so it's extra important that they are protected from damage. Physical damage from head injuries is an obvious issue that can have lasting impact, but it's the less obvious damage done by restrictions to blood flow into and through the brain, and by inflammation and oxidative stress that are the most likely contributors to dementia, as already discussed.

~ ~ ~

Eating foods that help keep your blood vessels in peak condition is essential. It's probable that it's mostly how they have fared in your early adulthood and middle life that is most important here, but it's never too late to help them out.

Glucose has been well covered elsewhere in this book but I'll cover others of importance here.

~ ~ ~

Fats, fatty acids, omega 3s

Fat is not always the bad guy it's been thought of for years. It's a normal component of many natural foods from meats, dairy foods, nuts, seeds, oils, grains, and some vegetables, and it carries many of the flavour components of foods. It gives foods a creamy mouth feel and importantly is great at keeping appetite up to scratch at a time in life when it is so easily challenged.

The marine omega 3 fats get a lot of interest and almost everyone seems to take one or other type of fish or krill oil. These contain the DHA and EPA that are found in high concentrations in the brain and have a variety of vital roles in cognitive function (as well as in other parts of the body – the heart most of all). There has been an abundance of the research work done on DHA especially and it is accepted as a powerful protector of brain cells. But it's most likely that all the omega-3s have important roles to play, which medical research has not yet completely identified, and relying on only one type may miss some benefits the others can provide. ALA it seems, may help your brain cells keep up fuel supplies, and EPA looks as if it may limit the production of β amyloid.

ALA has been thought of as a poor cousin to DHA and EPA because experiments in laboratories showed it didn't seem to be converted very well into the DHA the brain needs. Nevertheless, when scientists recently looked at the amount of DHA in the blood of people who had eaten lots of ALA but no DHA, they found there was plenty produced so it may not be so black and white after all.

Also, if fish oil were the answer many claim it to be to DHA levels in the brain and thus to cognitive capacity, then vegetarians who don't eat fish and vegans who eat no animal products at all would have very low levels and a greater chance of developing dementia. That's just not so – maybe their intake of ALA is providing more than was originally thought.

The danger of taking large amounts of anything is that it can unbalance other nutrients and when you take enough – the sorts of amounts many people take of fish oils at times – they act like a medication, not a nutrient and so can have side effects that may not be helpful. With Omega 3s, it is important to remember that they are also contributors to oxidation reactions in brain cells – remember oxidation is the way energy is produced so it's good but it's important to provide a balance so that excess oxidative wastes are not produced. That balance needs to come from antioxidant foods. It is hard to eat enough antioxidants to balance a very high dose of omega 3s in tablet form, so it's very important before taking any tablets, no matter how innocuous you think they might be, to check them with your doctor.

Interestingly the widely touted Mediterranean diet may well gain its plusses from the abundance of antioxidants it supplies from fruit, vegetables, legumes, and good quality olive oil along with the omega-3 and good protein from fish and seafood.

FOOD SOURCES OF OMEGA-3 FATS

ALA	flax seeds (linseed)
	walnuts and less in other nuts
	leafy green vegetables
	some oils, particularly canola
EPA and DHA	fish oil
(also called long chain omega-3s)	fish and other seafood, especially oily cold water fish like salmon, tuna, mackerel, and sardines
	grass fed meats and poultry
	wild meats (like kangaroo or rabbit)
	egg yolks
	the brain and liver of meat animals

~ ~ ~

The antioxidant vitamins: A, C, E

Vitamin A

Good Sources: butter, fortified margarines, organ meats, egg yolks, yellow and orange fruits and vegetables

This is not a vitamin you usually have to worry about, as it's rare to become deficient most of the time, but changes in the way it's handled in the body as you age can alter how much is available to brain cells. It is one of the antioxidant vitamins so has an important part to play in cell protection as well as in maintaining cognitive function. But it is stored in the liver and in body fat and they seem to accumulate it as you age, but also to hold onto it so it's not as available as it might be for its work in the brain. That means a regular intake is always important and in time research may well suggest a slightly higher amount is needed than is currently advised to compensate for inadequacies in retrieving what's been stored in body fat and the liver.

Fortunately, as long as you eat a good variety of vitamin A containing foods it's unusual to run into a deficiency. But because it accumulates in the liver, it is also important to avoid high doses in tablet form, (particularly as retinol above 3000 micrograms per day) as that may cause liver damage and even increase your risk of hip fracture.

This is definitely one you need to check with your doctor.

Vitamin C

Good Sources: citrus fruits, capsicum, and other peppers, cabbage

Other sources: leafy vegetables

Vitamin C acts directly as an antioxidant; it protects vitamin E and folate from degradation, and is needed to make neurotransmitters, so it's not surprising that low levels of this vitamin are also closely associated with reduced cognitive abilities.

There have been numerous claims made over the years about the benefits of taking high doses of this vitamin in tablet or powder form and most recently suggesting it can protect against dementia. But while it certainly is essential in that, it is unlikely to act in the same way when removed from its original food source. It's possible the many other substances that exist with it in those foods also have antioxidant properties and roles to play. It is likely that, when separated, they do not work as they originally did.

Supplements are useful when there are deficiencies but many other claims are probably commercially driven and possibly inflated.

Vitamin E

Good sources: nuts and seeds, and oils made from them, wheat germ, and egg yolk

Other sources: avocado, leafy vegetables

Vitamin E is one of the most powerful nutritional antioxidants. It promotes efficient blood flow through the brain and elsewhere and plays an important role in the immune defence system.

Science has found that people with low levels of vitamin E have poorer memory and lower cognitive abilities so many believe taking a supplement will boost their cognitive abilities. Sadly, that doesn't seem to work – again it may be a case of natural food providing the best source.

Deficiency is not very common, though it can happen when fat is not being absorbed properly as it is a fat-soluble vitamin. This can occur in some illnesses, and especially where there is chronic gastrointestinal upset.

When appetite is down and food intake is low however, this is one to ask your doctor about.

The other essential vitamins

Vitamin D

Good sources: the most important provider is that made under your skin when it is exposed to sunlight. Also pink fleshed fish (such as salmon and ocean trout), oily fish (mackerel, sardines), and cod liver oil.

Other sources: egg yolk, butter, fortified margarine, mushrooms that have had time in the sun (field grown) or have been irradiated with UV light (available in some stores and labelled as such). You can add vitamin D to any mushrooms, even those purchased in a supermarket, by putting them in the sun just for 5 or 10 minutes and they hold that until you eat them.

Deficiency of vitamin D is a big problem affecting up to one third of people in Australia and more likely in older age. In hostels and aged care facilities, that figure jumps to over half the residents!

Most people will know it's essential for bones, but it's far, far more than that. Insufficient vitamin D also causes weakness and pain in your large muscles, affecting walking. It contributes to heart disease, certain cancers (colorectal, breast, and prostate particularly) and diabetes and some other illnesses.

But while we don't yet know exactly how it works in the brain its role in there is undeniable because there are specific receptors within the brain for vitamin D and its metabolites. We know it is involved in plasticity, in the survival of neurones and in transmission of information and is thought to play a role in depression and anxiety – both, which of course also impact cognitive abilities either in the short or long term.

Unlike most vitamins, you only get small amounts of vitamin D from foods naturally, so most of what you need you produce yourself through your skin when you are in the sun. In our modern lives now that we don't get the same sun exposure our forebears did, we risk not getting enough vitamin D.

If you tend to be involved in mostly indoor activities, work indoors, find it difficult to get outside, or choose to avoid the sun for other reasons such as skin cancer concerns, then you are very likely not getting enough Vitamin D. If you are out and about every day, gardening, fishing, walking or doing other similar outdoor activities and exposing at least your arms and some of your legs and face without sunscreen for about half an hour most days, then you might be able to get what you need. But for anyone else and during winter especially, choosing foods with Vitamin D and adding supplements to make up any shortfall is the way to go.

If you are not sure, ask your doctor to arrange a blood test to have your vitamin D status assessed. If your levels are just a bit low, or if they are fine *but* you are not getting any sun, a low dose supplement each day is probably needed. If you are found to be deficient, you may need quite a lot more and it can take a few months to get those levels back up.

The B vitamins

Vitamin B1 (thiamine)

Good sources: fortified breakfast cereals.

Thiamine plays a vital role in neurotransmission, so is indispensable in the brain. We have no way of storing this vitamin so it must be eaten daily. It's fortunate then that it is found in many foods, but a deficiency can develop in people who drink excessive amounts of alcohol because it is also used in the detoxification of alcohol in the body.

Vitamin B3 (niacin)

Good sources: fortified breakfast cereals, nuts, meat, and whole grains.

Niacin, along with the other B group vitamins (thiamine B1 and riboflavin B2) is needed to make neurotransmitters. There are lots of claims around giving niacin wonder nutrient status for the brain and, more traditionally, for heart function. Unfortunately, many are inflated claims. Vitamin B3 is certainly essential to brain function and in some people is used therapeutically to assist in managing heart disease but only under strict medical supervision to avoid an excess causing other problems.

Although it's important to be sure to get enough B3, a deficiency is rare unless you have been eating poorly for quite some time, and then it will be only one of many nutrients lacking.

Vitamin B6

Good sources: eggplant (aubergine), fortified breakfast cereals and veal are highest, but B6 is found in a wide variety of foods including wholegrain breads and cereal foods, potatoes, nuts and seeds, meats, organ meats, fish, banana, and avocado.

B6 is important in assisting brain activity, but it also plays an integral part in regulating levels of homocysteine that is discussed in the text box here. In fact, B6 has recently been touted as helping to avoid Alzheimer's disease, partly because of its effect on homocysteine.

It's in lots of foods so deficiency is unusual but research is continuing around whether getting extra is a good or a bad thing... As with the other B vitamins of special importance to your brain, B6 is in many foods so the chances you'll miss out are similar to niacin.

A NOTE ON HOMOCYSTEINE

If you read a bit on health you may have heard mention of homocysteine and how it's bad for your heart and might cause stroke and Alzheimer's disease, and that is certainly true if the levels in your blood are too high.

But homocysteine in just the right amount has an important role to play too. It comes from the proteins we eat and, with the help of the vitamins folate, B6 and B12, is used to make two substances that are very good for you, one of which is a powerful antioxidant called glutathione.

It's only a problem when homocysteine doesn't get converted into glutathione, which happens if your levels of these B vitamins are too low, so it builds up in your blood. Keeping homocysteine levels just right depends on making sure you don't become deficient, but unfortunately taking extra vitamins beyond that doesn't add extra benefit You might hear some big claims made that various supplements reduce homocysteine levels, but always check with your doctor before taking these vitamins in tablet form. Taking them when you are not deficient can cause you harm.

You might also hear about supplements of glutathione itself with claims that it will help but, sadly, the reality is that these don't get absorbed well enough to be of much use, despite their considerable cost, so will probably give you little or no benefit.

Folate (sometimes called vitamin B9)

Good sources: darker green vegetables including kale, spinach, Asian vegetables, broccoli, liver, commercial breakfast cereals, and juices with added folate.

Other sources: nuts, chickpeas, and yeast, or vegetable extracts such as Vegemite and Marmite.

A deficiency of folate (also in foods as 'folic acid') is well known to cause cognitive decline. When levels of this vitamin are low in your body, your chances of developing Alzheimer's disease are significantly increased.

Luckily, folate is found in a lot of foods and if you eat well you'll usually be okay. Problems can crop up because some common medications interfere with the way folate is used in the body. (See the list here). If you take any of these medications for more than a week or so you should be having your folate status checked regularly by your doctor and may need supplements or other interventions if your levels are too low.

Take care though: don't take a folate supplement unless your doctor prescribes it. This is one vitamin you mustn't get too much of, because it can worsen kidney problems or hide the signs of a damaging vitamin B12 deficiency.

A mild deficiency of folate might set you on a path to heart or cognition problems. A severe deficiency can cause diarrhoea, loss of appetite, weight loss, weakness, sore tongue, headaches, heart palpitations, irritability, and forgetfulness.

The common NSAID (non-steroidal anti-inflammatory drug) pain relievers on the list of medications here, including ibuprofen and aspirin, are worth a special mention (not paracetamol — Panadol — which is a different type of pain relief medication). Because you can buy them at a supermarket or chemist without a prescription so many people believe them to be completely safe and may take them often enough to affect folate levels. If you do take them regularly without a script, let your doctor know. You may need to try alternative medications or take folate supplements if there is an issue. Other NSAIDs cause similar problems but are only available on prescription, and your doctor can easily monitor them.

Very low dose aspirin such as Cartia 100, Cardiprin 100 brands are often prescribed to help reduce the 'stickiness' in the blood and thus avoid heart attack and stroke. These low dose tablets don't cause the problems higher doses of most NSAIDs do, but your folate status should be monitored regularly if you take them routinely.

Before you think of taking folate as a tablet, a word of caution: get a test to check if you are deficient first, because getting too much folate on its own can also be harmful. Usually a blood test for folate will also check your vitamin B12 levels because these two vitamins are dependent on each other.

And be extra careful if you have reduced kidney function. Taking high doses of folate alone or in very high doses with other B vitamins in tablet form can worsen any kidney damage. While most lower dose combined-B vitamin supplements contain both folate and B12 in amounts that won't cause you harm, you must always discuss taking any vitamin or mineral supplement tablet with your doctor to avoid causing yourself extra problems.

MEDICATIONS WHICH MAY AFFECT FOLATE STATUS

(brand names in italics)

Metformin for diabetes	including *Diabex, Diaformin, Formet, Glucobet, Glucophage, Glucophage XR, Metex*
Sulphasalazine used in IBS, Crohn's disease and ulcerative colitis	including *Salazopyrin, Salazopyrin SR, Pyralin EN*
Phenytoin anticonvulsant / anti epileptic	*Dilantin*
Methotrexate used in cancer therapy and rheumatoid arthritis	*Methoblastin*
Triamterene, a diuretic	including *Hydrene 25/50*
Barbiturates (sedatives not often used nowadays)	Other names amylobarbitone and amobarbital
Some blood lipid lowering fibrates	Including: Fenofibrate (*Lipidil*)
Non-steroidal anti-inflammatory medications (NSAIDs) for mild or moderate pain, fever and inflammation relief	Available without prescription –including ibuprofen: *(Nurofen, Advil and generics)* naproxen (*Naprosyn*), and aspirin Others available only on prescription include: diclofenac (*Voltaren*), celecoxib (*Celebrex*), meloxicam (*Mobic*), piroxicam (*Feldene*), indomethacin (*Indocid*), mefanamic acid (*Ponstan*), ketoprofen (*Orudis*)

Vitamin B12

Good sources: animal foods of all types, especially meat

Other sources: fortified soy milk, yeast, and foods made with it (bread etc)

Vitamin B12 deficiency is worryingly common in older age and because it shares some symptoms with dementia is a particular concern, as you've already heard. B12 is essential for correct functioning of nerves and for making healthy blood cells, and a deficiency can cause confusion, difficulty concentrating, memory loss, irritability, depression, anaemia, fatigue, shortness of breath, tingling and numbness in the limbs, loss of balance and reduced appetite.

Luckily, prompt diagnosis and treatment can reverse all of these quickly so it's important to check with your doctor if you are worried. It would be a tragedy if permanent nerve or brain damage happens when it could have been avoided.

As with folate, most people should easily get enough B12 in their diet, but because we get B12 almost exclusively from animal foods, vegetarians or anyone, who eats limited amounts of animal foods, might struggle.

Despite it being available in foods, B12 deficiency becomes common as you get older because of age-related changes in your stomach and intestines that make you less able to absorb it. It needs just the right amount of acid from your stomach to allow it to be absorbed from the gut. But two things reduce those levels so that absorption also falls and over the years that can quite easily result in deficiency with disastrous consequences. Firstly, acid production in the stomach reduces as you get older and secondly, medication you might be taking for reflux reduces acid production further: there is a list in the text box here but it's most likely with the Proton Pump Inhibitors (PPIs). You must not stop taking your medication of course, but your B12 levels must be checked regularly if you have been on one of these for more than about 5 years. As well, if you suffer recurrent gastrointestinal upset or diarrhoea as you may in IBS, as a side effect of antibiotics or due to other illness, you can miss out on your B12.

Last, but certainly not least, if you gradually cut down on eating meat and other animal foods as you get older you set yourself up for a B12 deficiency.

B12 is also involved with folate in homocysteine conversion so a deficiency can cause higher levels of homocysteine in the blood. Check out more about homocysteine in the text box here.

If any of these issues apply to you, or if you take medications listed here, you need to have your B12 levels checked regularly. Correcting a deficiency is easily achieved with a regular injection so it's worth doing.

LIST OF COMMON ANTIREFLUX MEDICATIONS WHICH MAY AFFECT B12 LEVELS WHEN USED OVER A NUMBER OF YEARS

The PPIs (proton pump inhibitors):	**Esomeprazole** (*Nexium*)
	Lansoprazole (*Zoton*)
	Omeprazole (*Losec, Prohibitor*)
	Pantoprazole (*Somac*)
	Rabprazole (*Pariet*)
The H2 blockers are less likely to cause problems but also reduce stomach acid so having B12 status checked is prudent in late age	**Ranitidine** (*Zantac, Rani,Ranitidine*)
	Cimetidine (*Tagamet*)
	Nizatidine (*Tazac*)
	Famotidine (*Amfamox, Pepcidine*)

The Minerals

Iodine

Good sources: Found in high levels in seaweed, so anything that contains seaweed (nori) including sushi; also from most seafood, especially shellfish; and of course from foods prepared with iodised salt (salt that has had iodine added).

Iodine is vital for your thyroid function and is important for your brain health and keeping your body processes regulated. The amount of iodine that foods contain, depends on how much is in the soil, and in Australia, unfortunately, those levels are low. Years ago, iodine was commonly added to table salt to boost the amount people ate but now people often avoid salt or eat 'gourmet' salt (sea salt crystals, pink salt, etc.) which don't contain iodine. We also used to get a lot from milk and dairy foods but that came from iodine-based cleaning products used in dairies, a practice which is now out of favour, so dairy foods don't supply the iodine they once did.

It's likely many older people don't get enough iodine and that can be damaging for your brain. Making sure the salt you use is iodised is important.

Iron

Good sources: red meats, liver, kidney are the highest; followed by pork, poultry, and seafood.

Other sources: soy foods, lentils, spinach, seeds, and fortified breakfast cereals.

Most people know that you become anaemic if your iron levels fall too low, but what you may not know is that a mild iron deficiency, which isn't even obvious without a blood test, can contribute to reduced cognition. Iron is needed to make neurotransmitters, helps in the protection of brain cells, and supplies them with indispensable oxygen.

Moreover, because the brain does so much, its oxygen needs are high so even a minor shortfall means it can't function properly. If that shortfall continues, permanent damage happens.

Three things can set you up for iron deficiency. Firstly, medical conditions which cause you to lose blood (e.g. from chronic ulcers in your stomach or upper intestine, anything which causes blood loss from the bowel — including bowel cancer— bleeding gums, or frequent cuts, bruises, and grazes). Secondly, any medical issue or medication that reduces your ability to absorb iron from food. Lastly, but certainly not least because it's so very common, gradually cutting down on eating high iron foods like red meat.

Iron, like vitamin B12, needs stomach acid for efficient absorption and you have read how that declines with age and medications. Surprisingly, some food and drinks make it more difficult to get iron from your meals. Tea is one, so, as you get older, it's very important to avoid drinking tea with your meals. Leave at least an hour between eating a meal and having your cup of tea (that doesn't apply to green tea, herbal tea, infusions or coffee).

It can take many months or years for your iron levels to get low enough to cause even a mild deficiency but if any of the above are familiar to you, make sure you have regular blood tests.

Prevention is, as always, prudent. From now on, make sure you get iron-containing foods a few days a week: liver (lambs fry), kidney, red meats, poultry and fish, are the best sources so vegetarians especially should be vigilant. If you know your levels are low a bit extra is a good idea.

But you may have read recently about iron accumulating in brain cells and contributing to dementia so that needs looking at here also.

First, let me be absolutely clear: iron is essential for the formation of neurotransmitters in the brain and inadequate levels in the brain are thought to be involved in things like ADHD so clearly it is vital in brain health. However, it does accumulate in the brain in everyone as we age so it's not unusual. But is it a problem? It depends on what causes it and unfortunately, we don't exactly know. But one contributor may be what has been left behind after a so-called micro-bleed in the brain. This is a tiny area somewhat like a stroke but far, far smaller where a tiny blood vessel 'bursts' and bleeds, causing blood supply to areas of the brain nearby to be deprived of resources. These are often hardly noticeable to those who have them, but they leave behind some iron even when bleeding has stopped and repairs have been done. These events individually, like TIAs, may have little long-term effect for quite some time, especially as plasticity accommodates issues that may arise in healthy, active people. However, over time they can add up until they contribute to cognitive decline and dementia.

ZINC, IRON AND COPPER ACCUMULATION AND DEMENTIA

Recent research has shown that unusual accumulation of all of these minerals in the brain causes severe problems that can lead to dementia. These include accelerating accumulation of β amyloid, increased oxidative stress, and disruption of the working of the blood brain barrier and cell death.

But these nutrients are also essential for all sorts of functions throughout the body and brain and deficiencies of all can be devastating.

So it comes down to balance and the long-term cell protection from antioxidants, anti-inflammatory foods and possibly carnosine that is covered in Chapter 2.

When you get mineral nutrients from foods, they come with a wide variety of other substances that probably assist the body to use them well, and if they are eaten as part of a meal with other different foods that helps too. If, in contrast they are taken in tablet form without a diagnosed deficiency, no matter how plausible the promotional information that accompanies that product, they are far more likely to cause imbalances that the body can't accommodate. Protecting brain cells from the damaging effects of inflammation and oxidation, probably helps avoid the imbalance that causes these minerals to build up unnaturally.

But before everyone gives up meat, which of course is a valuable source of protein and a range of other essential nutrients as well as iron, it looks like this is about more than just whether you eat foods containing iron or not. It seems that there is something going wrong that causes the usual balancing of iron in the brain to be upset, rather than that iron is toxic in any way in the normal amounts eaten in foods. Certainly, there is always a risk in taking supplements: even multivitamin/mineral tablets can cause an excess intake of iron or copper if you are also eating reasonably well. These minerals are needed in just the right amounts and the body is far better at dealing with them when they are in food and accompanied with all the things they usually go along with, than given in a synthetic form without all those things. Too little iron is sure to reduce cognition, too much may well also but that's most likely when you are not deficient and it's taken in tablet form or you eat very high iron foods – liver, kidney or wild meats like venison– often without the balance of plenty of vegetables, grains, and other foods. If you are in doubt, ask your doctor to check your iron levels, and then decide what is best for you.

~ ~ ~

There is an inherited disorder called haemochromatosis (or hemochromatosis) where iron builds up in the body potentially causing damage to many cells and people are encouraged to reduce iron from food, but this is not relevant in this discussion.

~ ~ ~

Getting a wide variety of foods is always the key to balance but I see no need for those who enjoy red meat to give it up, just enjoy a variety of protein foods.

Zinc

Good sources: oysters are far higher than any other food, also red meats, and wild meats, a bit less in pork, chicken, and fish.

Other sources: fortified breakfast cereals (ie: zinc added during manufacture), nuts, seeds, honey, and maple syrup.

Zinc is second only to iron in content in the brain and has vital roles in creating and maintaining brain cells and in neurotransmission.

People who don't get enough of it suffer from reduced memory, learning ability, and cognition. But get too much, and a bit like iron, it seems it might play a part in the development of dementia by contributing to accumulation of β amyloid so balance is absolutely essential.

It's fortunate that getting too much from food is unlikely unless you eat nothing but oysters all the time because they happen to be very high in zinc!

What's most likely again is overzealous intake of supplements or tablets containing zinc: these might be taken with the intention of helping in things like wound healing, fighting infections, improving your sense of taste or your appetite, or along with other nutrients like vitamin C, vitamin E, and beta-carotene to help avoid macular degeneration. Even though zinc is important for all those things, it's only needed in small amounts, and unless you are actually deficient, taking more than is needed could cause you problems. More is not better with nutrient minerals no matter what the marketing might say. Even those multivitamin/mineral tablets, if taken when you don't really need them can contribute, so always check with your doctor. You only need to take higher dose tablets when you know you are deficient to get your levels up to where they should be.

Like iron, your body accesses and regulates zinc best when you get it from animal foods so; again, vegetarians need to be more careful.

Magnesium

Main sources: Soy beans and soy foods, nuts and nut butters, seeds, rice, wheat bran, whole grains and foods made with them, molasses, treacle, dark sugars (dark brown sugar and similar), corn, corn products, and maize products

Contain less but useful additions: dark green vegetables, sun dried tomatoes, milk powder, and fish.

Magnesium is a remarkable nutrient, active in a huge number of body processes. It's important in coordinating muscle contraction, nerve transmission, maintaining the rhythm of your heart, producing healthy bone, releasing energy from food, building protein for muscle tissue, and assisting with blood glucose control. It is also extremely important to the brain.

There are all sorts of ways magnesium can contribute to cognitive decline: an inadequate intake reduces the removal of β amyloid and increases chronic inflammation and oxidative stress all of which of course contribute to Alzheimer's. It has lots of roles in enzyme systems throughout the body and brain and is essential in muscle activity and strength. Perhaps most importantly in the brain day by day, it helps in the release of neurotransmitters and is absolutely vital to the work of the mitochondria, which are the power supply systems in each cell, so any issues with its availability very quickly affect the brain's capacity to do any task.

Magnesium faces two problems: the first is to do with changed eating habits and food processing. It's a mineral that is concentrated in the outer layers of grains and in less refined foods so our modern diet tends to provide less than it once did. It also needs to be available in the soil to get into vegetables so unless vegetables are grown in a good soil they can be low in magnesium. Stick with whole grain foods for their fibre and add some soy products, nuts and seeds, and you will get magnesium too.

The second problem has to do with how well it is retained in the body. Unfortunately, even if it's in food, magnesium gets more difficult to absorb with age. That's because of changes in the ability of the gut to absorb it as well as the effects of medications including diuretics (common brand names in Australia are *Frusemide*, *Lasix* and *Microzide*) and some antibiotics, as well as the increased tendency of the kidneys to pass it out in the urine. It is thought that Vitamin D helps in its absorption, so if that is low, getting enough can have added challenges.

It's another one to take care with if you are considering a supplement because higher doses cause diarrhoea. (In fact, *Milk of Magnesia* is an old-fashioned cure all for indigestion and constipation - it contains magnesium hydroxide and is an osmotic laxative, and *Epsom salt* is magnesium sulfate and works the same way if you consume it, instead of putting it in your bath). Lower dose tablets are usually fine but again always check with your doctor as it can interact with some medications.

Selenium

Good sources: nuts (especially Brazil nuts) fish, seafood, liver, kidney, red meat, chicken, eggs, mushrooms, and grains. (The level of selenium in foods usually depends on how much is in the soil from which they are sourced.).

Selenium is a powerful antioxidant that protects brain cells as well as bolstering the effects of some other antioxidant substances including vitamin C.

It's made health news in recent years with the discovery that people who have better selenium status have better brain health and the possibility that it also helps fight some cancers, especially prostate cancer. The understandable desire to avoid prostate cancer might lead some people to take large amounts of selenium but unfortunately getting too much is just as much a problem as too little because it's toxic in high doses.

If you are concerned that you might not be getting enough, always get your doctor to check your selenium status but getting it from food presents few problems.

All minerals and most vitamins are best coming from food — the amounts foods contain are not excessively high and you get the benefit of the variety of other nutrients those foods also contain.

WHAT'S THE LATEST ABOUT SALT IN FOODS?

Processing food by adding salt (everyday salt contains sodium and that's what is significant) in the past when refrigeration was inadequate or less widely available was an extremely important way of keeping food for as long as possible. But we got used to that flavour and anyone who grew up eating salted meat and other foods preserved with salt will attest to its appeal. That doesn't mean those are bad foods it just means that more and more we need balance: the foods that have salt and to some extent sugars added for their preservation and taste appeals with fresh fruits, vegetables, nuts, seeds, meat, and dairy foods that are naturally low in salt.

Nowadays food processing often adds salt to accommodate the taste requirements of consumers, so eating an excessive amount of foods that have undergone processing from their original form can add to the salt load in the body. But, is that a problem?

For many years advice has consistently advocated a low salt diet for a range of health benefits, but a recent wide-ranging review of the evidence by the Institute of Medicine in the US (an independent collaboration of research experts) found that both very high and low levels were problematic. What was more significant than sodium (in regular salt) however was the potassium you eat. It seems as long as your potassium intake is good, it is less important how much sodium you get.

And as potassium is found in many foods – especially fruits and vegetables – there are benefits to eating extra potassium because of the antioxidants these foods also contain. (See the list below)

The thing about enjoying the salt taste is that the more salt you eat, the more you need in order to enjoy foods in the same way. If you cut down, you need to do it gradually so you get used to the change and your enjoyment continues.

But remember that your taste ability unfortunately, declines with age so you might actually need more salt or other flavours in foods to be able to appreciate them as you always have. If food tastes like nothing and that means you find it a challenge to eat at all then adding salt to foods might be what's needed to ward off malnutrition. It's always a balance, and it's always a matter for each individual to consider quality of life and weigh up what's really important.

For anyone already living with dementia it may be that adding extra salt to food to encourage intake and enjoyment and avoid the far more dangerous problems that weight loss can cause might just be the answer – add potassium-containing foods where possible to give an extra benefit.

Foods high in potassium: most yellow or orange fruits (particularly bananas) and vegies, tomatoes, legumes, lentils and dried beans of all types, broccoli, kale, Brussel sprouts, dried fruits, milk and dairy foods, nuts and seeds, and chocolate.

Chapter 5

TOO FAT? TOO THIN? – PUTTING BODY WEIGHT INTO PERSPECTIVE IN DEMENTIA

Before we look at the ins and outs of how your bodyweight influences your chances of developing dementia, let's get one thing straight:

Nothing beats activity and exercise for boosting brain as well as body health to keep you independent in the years ahead: it doesn't matter how big or how small you are, exercise is a non-negotiable necessity because it's far more powerful in protecting your brain than any food or diet.

Now that's settled, let's talk about what you should weigh and why.

Surely, obesity is bad for your health.

Yes it is. Obesity in younger age sets you up for all sorts of health issues: diabetes, cardiovascular disease, issues with your joints and a range of other concerns not the least of which is cognitive decline. In fact, obesity in younger and middle age might triple your chance of developing dementia later in age! There is a grim truth here though: many people who have been obese throughout their lives don't actually make it into their 80s. But if that hasn't been the case, then maybe you have a genetic advantage over others and that's an area of study where the surface has only been scratched so far. Whatever the reason, the time to lose excess weight is well before your late 60s.

As I have said many times and will be discussed later in this chapter, once you are in your late 60s or beyond, while weight loss might be helpful to reduce strain on your joints or to reduce your risk of cardiovascular issues, help your diabetes or just make life easier, it cannot safely be achieved by dieting or anything that focuses *only* on reducing the food your body and brain get (such as weight loss surgery), unless there is a very good exercise component along with a high protein diet to avoid muscle loss. Sure, you might lose plenty of weight and that looks good on the scales, but a lot of that will be muscle loss that you can't see and losing that will do you far more harm than the excess body fat you had previously.

It's important to remember that most public health messages advocating weight loss diets are fine for people in their 30s, 40s, 50s, even early 60s as long as exercise is included, but they can be anything from unhelpful to damaging if you are instead closer to 80 or 90. Unfortunately, it's too often older people who are heeding these messages when they are really for those far younger.

For anyone who is now in their late 70s or beyond, most of you are at a decided advantage cognition-wise because you grew up when life was less sedentary. We are designed to be physically active our entire lives – so many of the ills of ageing stem from us doing less than we should day in, day out. Kids need to be out playing, running, climbing, enjoying sports; that necessity doesn't change just because you got older. You got to be a child in the days before life was so sedentary – you probably walked to school, often long distances; were shooed outside to play every spare minute, and had plenty of labour intensive chores to do each day. If you have gained some kilos into your 70s, as long as you have remained active they are probably doing you good.

If you have always been lean, you don't need to rush out to try to gain weight. Just stop listening to advice suitable for 30 and 40 year olds that suggests thin is ideal —science begs to differ for you now: instead, gaining a few kilos could even be your best advice.

For anyone not yet in their late 60s or beyond there isn't a moment to wait: combining exercise and activity reduces excess bodyweight, improves the actions of insulin (reducing insulin resistance), and reduces oxidative stress and inflammation when you need it most to help cheat dementia.

Just don't take up the latest 'get thin quick' regime.

So what is it about obesity that contributes to dementia?

You'd think that obesity is just about eating more calories than you use up, and that's most of the story. There is a little bit more to the picture that ends up impacting cognition: that's the fact that eating just a bit more food than the body needs day in, day out (called chronic overnutrition by nutritional scientists) not only adds to body fat stores but it also creates oxidative stress and inflammation in the brain. Now here is where it gets interesting – both oxidative stress and inflammation affect cognition directly, but they also can cause disruption in the energy regulation systems in the brain. That triggers messages of hunger or a need to eat when it's not really necessary, which leads to overnutrition and weight gain, in turn increasing oxidative stress and inflammation, so the cycle continues...

As you read in Chapter 3, oxidative damage (to which oxidative stress is a contributor) and inflammation are drivers of cognitive decline and contribute to the accumulation of β amyloid and tau proteins. For the health of your brain, anyone in younger or middle age who is obese or overweight must do all they can to lose excess weight *before* later age.

The solution lies in getting plenty of exercise and activity to reduce the stress and inflammation, and in cutting down food intake, or perhaps using an intermittent fasting technique (a couple of days a week eating very little, then the rest of the week eating normally) to help out. Even if you don't achieve lots of weight loss, exercise and activity are essential for your brain.

But as has been said many times in this book and my former one, things are not the same in later age. Inactivity and sedentary lifestyles do so often go along with obesity and they continue to impact inflammation and oxidative damage. They also affect fuel supply to brain cells, reducing their ability to adapt and regenerate to counter any damage that does occur (in other words, their 'plasticity' is reduced). Doing everything you can to stop that happening by getting up, getting out and about, dancing, playing, going to the gym – whatever you can do and ideally adding more as you get fitter – is the answer now.

~ ~ ~

The problem of underweight in dementia

In dementia, especially Alzheimer's disease, weight loss, and underweight are far more likely to be the problems than overweight. In fact, around half of all people diagnosed have already unintentionally lost weight by then and if that is not dealt with quickly, it makes things so much worse – physically and mentally.

Turning weight loss around and encouraging food intake that helps body and soul can have many challenges in dementia, but it's undeniably important. Too often it is either disregarded, forgotten in the array of other things to be arranged or managed soon after diagnosis, or even worse is considered to be 'usual' and thus ignored. But it is one thing that can make so much difference to quality of life as well as having so many health spin-offs – reducing the risk of illness, infections and the chance of falls, while assisting with cognition.

It might seem obvious that weight loss in dementia or in the lead up to it is caused by people not eating enough. Food intake is challenged in dementia in many ways, including through swallowing problems, or lost connections between neurones that make negotiating the complex processes of buying and storing food, preparing it, and then negotiating cutlery or the social mores of the table to get it in. Eating can be a much bigger challenge than most could imagine.

But for the most part, those things occur after diagnosis when the illness has progressed somewhat. Weight loss occurs before then, when there probably have been only a few, if any, indicators that something was amiss. *Any* unintentional weight loss at later age is always something to have checked out –dementia may not be part of the picture at all, but if it is, early diagnosis provides access to new treatments and strategies that can slow its progress and boost the quality of life. Leave it, and you risk missing out on those as well as having to confront all the negative health consequences of weight loss in later age.

Weight loss in dementia is not all about eating less food. In fact, it's often the opposite: *more* food can be being eaten or things remain apparently the same as usual but there is obvious weight loss. We know now that dementia seems to cause the body to expend more energy than is usual, so extra food is needed just to stay the same.

This is an intriguing finding and it probably explains why people have already lost weight by the time other symptoms have become obvious enough to result in a diagnosis. It has always been known that unexplained weight loss can be a sign things are awry and can herald undiagnosed physical illness like cancer, but it's now clear that it could also be a sign of cognitive decline.

It has to involve a change in one or all of the three ways that energy is expended in the body – an increase in basal metabolic rate, an increase in the energy used to maintain body temperature, or extra physical activity.

If you ask most people what is the biggest contributor to energy expenditure in the body they would say exercise – it seems logical and it's so obvious when you sweat and pant and get hot that something is going on in the body. But while it certainly has a significant impact during activity, it's the basal metabolic rate (BMR) that actually uses more most of the time. The BMR is the energy used up doing all the things needed to keep us alive, to keep cells and organs functioning, the heart beating, the lungs pumping, and significantly to keep that energy hungry brain working. Most of the time, it accounts for around three-quarters of the energy the body uses.

Additionally, a lot of energy is expended to keep the temperature of the body just right. Sweating to cool down and shivering to warm up both use much more than you might imagine.

The extra used when you exercise can be huge, but it's not usually that alone making the difference in the lead up, to or following diagnosis of dementia.

It's probably a combination of all three: a slightly higher BMR, problems with temperature regulation using more than usual to keep things on track, and increased activity. The latter is not usually extra gym workouts, but the combined effect of things like fidgeting, pacing, being uninclined to sit still, wandering, and repetitive behaviours.

This altered energy balance control is probably the result, like dementia, of the accumulated oxidative, inflammatory and blood flow related damage to the brain over many years – combined with a genetic potential yet to be clearly defined. Each of those bits of 'damage' would have been so inconsequential individually that there is no way to be sure if you had eaten all your greens as your mum advised, or avoided working in that factory, or not had that concussion, or had eaten more nuts or less chips, or played more or less sport, whether you might have avoided dementia. Those questions once you are in later age are pointless and unhelpful. The genetic research is mounting that different people are affected by different things by virtue of their genes but there is a still a way to go till we can use that knowledge to guide our choices. For now, it's a matter of doing what you can from where you are.

Anyone who cares for or about someone who is living with dementia needs to be aware that person will mostly feel just as hungry as always and appreciate good food as before. The issues are more with having the brain connections working well enough to communicate those things to others appropriately to ask for or accept food, and eventually the complexities of food preparation and eating might become difficult to manage also.

It is so important also to try not to restrict food. It might be hard to avoid when someone you care about starts to eat more food than usual, especially if its things that might be considered 'junk' – foods high in sugars, salt and fats, but unless they are gaining lots of weight, trying to reduce those foods might instead increase the chance of damaging weight loss. Always remembering to watch for changes in the way clothes fit is one good idea.

Of course just because someone begins to eat more food, that is no reason at all to suspect dementia. But if that is happening yet weight is obviously reducing, it's something that needs medical investigation. In some sorts of dementia (especially frontotemporal dementia - FTD) very excessive food intake may occur and cause a marked weight increase that makes getting about more difficult and can worsen issues like diabetes, increasing the complexity of the way it's managed. However, in most dementias, especially Alzheimer's and eventually too in FTD, weight loss is more of a problem so food restriction is to be avoided.

~ ~ ~

So what is the ideal weight for your brain at later age?

Again it's those who remain physically active in life and who exercise who also have the best cognition. But beyond that, among the wide range of shapes and sizes you see in older people, on average it's those who are a bit heavier who seem to have the advantage (at the higher end of the weight charts with a Body Mass Index or BMI, around 27 or even a bit higher). They tend to have better brain function and live longer than those who are much thinner (at the lower end of the chart with a BMI below 22). Most research now agrees that a BMI between 23 and 29 is best for older adults (as compared to 19 to 25 usually recommended for those 18+)

Who knows why this is? Maybe those who are heavier are that way because they have been eating more food and getting the benefit of extra nutrients. It could also be because, perhaps surprisingly, fat actually does something other than just boost cuddliness. Body fat cells produce very small amounts of hormones including one called leptin that helps regulate cognitive processes (as well as food intake, bone formation, and body temperature control), and is important in memory, learning, and in plasticity. Plasticity allows new connections to form if damage has affected functions in some parts of the brain so it can help reduce the impact of dementia by recruiting undamaged parts of the brain network to help where there are problems. Oestrogen is another hormone produced in adipose (fat) tissue that is thought to assist cognition.

There is also the fact that cuddliness is of course more than just body fat, it's also muscle and bone and body fluid. Weight loss will always involve losing some of all of these – it's just the proportions that change, with muscle loss making up a higher amount of that with increasing age. So while you might hope for and even be convinced by the scales that it's body fat that has gone, muscle will always have gone along with that. The fluids held in the lost muscle go too, contributing to dehydration, which, as already discussed, is bad for cognition.

Maybe the fact that healthy people tend to gain a bit of weight as they age (especially around the middle) is not so much the disaster it's so often made out to be, but instead is the body protecting itself from frailty. For anyone with dementia this might be even more important because being physically frail can so easily make continuing to live at home very much more challenging. In the early stages of dementia, it's quite possible to deal with various behaviour and cognitive changes while continuing to live much the same as previously. However, physical incapacity brings in a whole new set of challenges that can easily mean a move into assisted care is required prematurely. Avoiding weight loss as much as possible is essential to help maintain physical as well as mental capabilities.

That can mean thinking outside the health messages you have been trying to stick with for years. Protein and colours are just as important, but making sure there are plenty of treat foods to go with them (or to hide them!) that can be just as important. The good thing about fats and carbohydrates being eaten along with protein is that the protein won't be wasted being used up as fuel when they accompany it so there will be more protein available to do the things it really is needed for.

Whatever the reason, if you are already in your late 60s or older – dementia or not - the message is clear: if you are just a bit cuddly, it's probably not a bad thing for your brain.

~ ~ ~

What about Calorie Restriction or Intermittent Fasting?

You may have read about or heard talk that calorie restriction or intermittent fasting — not eating at all on one or more days a week, (included in the 5/2 *plan* and similar diets) — can improve the health of your brain and also possibly extend your lifespan. In *Eat To Cheat Ageing* I touched on this in regard to what constitutes a health weight in later age and there I concluded that these regimes are, like most widely publicised diets, not for most people now in their seventies and beyond. That's because, at later age it's just not as simple as restricting any food intake on a couple of days a week then eating what you like on the others, as is mostly advised for younger people.

However, if you practice some sort of calorie restriction (short periods of little or no food intake without necessarily causing weight loss) when you are younger it may well assist with cognition later in life by reducing the inflammation caused by overnutrition.

Some recent research using rats found that calorie restriction might help brain cells use ketones to assist in fuel supply when glucose use is low. Whether this applies in humans is certainly not clear yet but in any case, it would apply to long-term restriction, as close as possible to lifelong. If you are now in your 60s or earlier, it may be worth a try, but only when the following are also part of the picture:

- a highly nutritious, protein and nutrient-dense diet that also restricts energy is eaten (this will require a very good understanding of nutrition)

- a well-planned exercise schedule to avert muscle loss, preferably also avoiding weight loss is involved

- weight loss should not be the aim – it is weight maintenance that is essential, even if you consider yourself overweight, (because the possible damage that losing body muscle could do likely outweighs any potential cognitive benefits).

The really good news from the research is that the exercise does the same sorts of things for your brain that periods of reduced food also do, so the importance of getting the exercise recommended throughout this and the previous book cannot be understated. For those who are able to take on incorporating periods of reduced food intake (without losing muscle) as well, that's a bonus. But for everyone else, there is no substitute for exercise and activity. Both exercise and intermittent food restriction increase the efficiency of fuel use by brain cells and both reduce excessive inflammation and oxidative stress on cells. Exercise does so much more than just make you feel 'fit', it provides your brain with powerful protective and support systems.

Chapter 6

DIABETES AND DEMENTIA

It's just one of the mysteries in dementia that glucose use within the brain is lowered very early in its development, well before diagnosis. And with the brain being such an energy powerhouse and thus needing so much more glucose to fuel its activities than the rest of the body, it's really not surprising that can have significant effects. The lower glucose use happens in people with diabetes and without it, but cognitive decline and dementia are also more common in people with diabetes. However, there is a bit of a chicken and egg scenario here – it's not entirely clear yet whether the reduced glucose use is specifically caused by problems with diabetes, or if it's diabetes-related issues that cause less glucose to be used.

But before we look further at this and before you despair, remember that everything already said about being active and eating to support your muscles and brain holds extra sway here. In fact, exercise is the ultimate weapon; having a good muscle reserve and staying active is a powerful regulator of blood glucose as well as insulin levels, so

SUGAR OR GLUCOSE?

Glucose is also called blood sugar but don't confuse it with sugar found in food.

All carbohydrate foods, including sugars as well as starches (such as found in grains and foods made from them and starchy vegetables) can be converted into glucose by digestion, which is then absorbed into the blood for distribution to all body cells where it can be used as fuel.

Sugars you might find in ingredient lists include glucose, fructose, concentrated fruit juice, high fructose corn syrup, maltose, maltodextrin, white, raw or brown sugar, honey, maple syrup, golden syrup, and treacle.

reduces the chances damage gets done in the brain. From your late 60s on, putting protein at the centre of every meal to support muscle while doing the activity and exercise you need, and combining that with getting those antioxidant rich, coloured and anti-inflammatory foods discussed elsewhere in this book will do so much to keep cognitive decline at bay – diabetes or not.

But as far as diabetes management goes, everything you already know is good, holds true for your brain also. Doing all you can to keep blood glucose levels as close as possible to those that occur without diabetes is key. And of course the extra benefit of staying active is that it helps keep damage to your heart and blood vessels that can reduce or block blood flow through the brain, at bay.

The effect of the glucose balancing act

The smooth running of the brain relies on a constant supply of glucose from the blood because it neither makes nor stores it itself. Even when ketones are also being used as discussed in Chapter 2, glucose always remains the predominant brain fuel. But like many things that appear 'simple,' achieving that relies on a complex interplay of many background processes. In the case of glucose, having just the right amount available keeps cells working as they should while either too much (*hyper*glycaemia) or too little (*hypo*glycaemia) causes problems for both body and brain.

The glucose balancing act- hypoglycaemia (low blood glucose)

It stands to reason that hypoglycaemia will challenge your ability to think and function because when that happens, fuel supply to the brain is severely impacted. This is obvious really, when it causes things like confusion, incoordination, blurred vision, and the like, (the basics of diabetes and ageing as well as day-to-day management strategies are covered in more detail in *Eat To Cheat Ageing*). In fact severe hypoglycaemia – especially in later age - can cause brain cell death and have far reaching health consequences, not the least of which of course is falling due to losing consciousness. I'll come back to the special considerations of diabetes at advanced age later in this chapter.

But the effects of more *mild* hypoglycaemia can be different: when you are young it seems that repeated episodes of mild hypoglycaemia that tend to occur occasionally when blood glucose control is 'tight' may actually induce some sort of adaptation by brain cells that is beneficial to cognition. That's great because long-term diabetes management guidelines for younger adults advocate this 'tight' control.

But when you have had diabetes a long time or it's been diagnosed in later years and you are now in your 70s or beyond, repeated episodes of hypoglycaemia, which of course means repeated episodes of undersupply of fuel to brain cells, is more likely instead to reduce cognition and possibly contribute to dementia. Unfortunately more severe hypos can become more common because at later age, they come on more quickly and the ability to recognise the usual warning signs is reduced.

The glucose balancing act – hyperglycaemia (high blood glucose)

When it comes to hyperglycaemia, an excess of glucose circulating in the blood might logically suggest extra fuel for brain activity and therefore boosted cognition. Sadly, though it's quite the opposite.

Blood glucose levels above what people without diabetes would have, instead increase the production of oxidative wastes, increase inflammation, cause the accumulation of toxic advanced glycation end products (AGEs), and upset the fine balance in a number of important systems in the brain. The result is damage to tiny blood vessels in the brain and accumulation of β amyloid and altered tau protein.

AGEs are a combination of glucose with some otherwise harmless things like protein fragments. But when they combine they become toxic to brain cells and unless they are whisked away quickly, they can do harm. They are produced in all of us as we age but diabetes both increases the likelihood of that and reduces the ability of the brain to clear them away so makes the chance of harm higher. AGEs increase oxidative stress as well as contributing more directly to the accumulation of β amyloid and other damaging substances.

I should mention here that AGEs can also be produced by cooking – mostly when protein foods like meats are cooked hot and dry as happens on a barbecue. Slower, moist cooking and not choosing 'well done' meats all the time reduces the amount you might eat. The effects of AGEs when eaten aren't the same as AGEs produced in the body in diabetes, but some researchers suggest that they can be harmful if eaten to excess. So again, variety in food intake remains the answer – not too much of any one food and get plenty of different colours to boost antioxidants for cell protection.

Staying on the straight and narrow

Not only do both high and low blood glucose present problems, but also the brain thrives on glucose levels in the blood (and therefore its glucose supply) staying as constant and predictable as possible: not swinging between too high and too low. In people without diabetes, insulin is able to automatically react to small changes in blood glucose levels, so they achieve the constancy the brain enjoys - always staying within a fairly tight range without ever going too high or too low. That is what diabetes management aims to mimic to avoid the well-recognised diabetes 'complications' affecting other organs like the heart, kidneys, and eyes. And smooth sailing – avoiding big fluctuations outside that tight range – is now thought to be of prime importance in keeping the brain healthy.

That's because, when blood glucose levels fluctuate a lot with bigger highs and smaller lows during the day occurring regularly, that triggers inflammation that you know by now is one of the main drivers of cognitive decline.

Those high/low swings can happen for all sorts of reasons but two are common in older people. Firstly, over-adjusting by eating too much extra carbohydrate after a hypo (whether mild or severe), so that levels swing from low to high quite quickly. Secondly, there is an understandable concern about the dangers of a hypo causing a fall as age advances so overly enthusiastic prevention strategies (eating extra carbohydrate) can inadvertently bring about big peaks.

A mention of the significance of diabetes-related blood vessel issues

Anything that slows or restricts blood flow into or through the brain hampers its function, increases inflammation in brain cells, and reduces the capacity to remove waste products and any other potentially damaging substances, including β amyloid.

It's well known that having diabetes means a higher risk of blockage in small blood vessels and that includes those in the brain. It's not surprising that even very small areas of restriction or blockage might cause tiny amounts of damage that add up over time, but restrictions in blood flow also contribute to inflammation and oxidative stress, compounding the issue. In all forms of diabetes including insulin resistance elevated blood pressure, elevated blood cholesterol, and the accumulation of excess body fat in the abdomen in early and middle age contribute to these issues in the brain, possibly more than we have realised in the past.

Everything you already do to keep the complications of diabetes at bay are the answers here too. That's especially true of activity and exercise; there is no substitute for the benefits they provide for body and brain.

The effect of elevated insulin levels

Both insulin resistance and type 2 diabetes increase insulin levels in the blood. That is because extra is needed due to cells throughout the body being less able to respond to insulin, so the pancreas delivers extra into the blood to compensate. There are also a number of substances associated with insulin including IGF (insulin-like growth factor) and many others that are among what I have called here insulin's 'associates' because they have roles in regulating blood and brain glucose alongside insulin. I'm not going to discuss them all here, but when I do look at insulin, do understand that some of these 'associates' may also be involved.

In the past the talk in diabetes management and the focus of most research was all on blood glucose, but more recently advances in medical technology have given us a better understanding of insulin itself and what it (often along with its associates) is doing in the brains of people with diabetes or insulin resistance.

When it comes to cognition, insulin has some extra and vital roles in the brain unrelated to its association with glucose, it assists with learning and the formation of memories, and helps regulate a number of neurotransmitters. As well, along with some 'associates,' it assists in plasticity of neurones and other cognitive functions. But to do any of those things it's needed in just the right amount.

If brain insulin levels are too low then so may be some neurotransmitters, there is likely to be a struggle to learn and form memories, and the brain's ability to adapt to localised damage through plasticity will be reduced.

But when blood insulin levels are higher than 'just right' there are a number of longer-term consequences that can contribute to dementia. High insulin levels increase inflammation (in both body and brain) with its brain-toxic consequences.

Also insulin, like all substances in the brain (be they vital to its function or waste products) needs to be removed to maintain those levels at 'just right.' The system that breaks insulin down for removal happens to do that also for β amyloid and here's where problems occur: insulin gets preferential treatment over β amyloid so if insulin levels are high removal of β amyloid slows down and the chance of β amyloid plaque forming increases.

As well, changes in the way many of insulin's associates work increases the chance that tau 'tangles' will develop.

Of course, if blood glucose levels are also high (as can occur in type 2 diabetes if not well managed) there is a double effect.

You can clearly see the problem elevated insulin levels pose for the brain but at the risk of broken record accusations – maintaining a good muscle reserve and keeping it working with activity and exercise will always help, mostly by reducing insulin resistance and thus body insulin levels.

The extra impact of accumulated body fat in the picture

The majority of people who are carrying excess body fat around their abdomen are also likely to be insulin resistant, whether they know it or not. And unfortunately when insulin resistance and excess body fat combine that amplifies the problems described above. Adipose (body fat) tissue is not an inert storage depot, it does things – some useful, some not. In later age a bit of extra body fat helps stave off frailty and assists cognition by producing tiny amounts of some hormones. But in early or middle age (when there are plenty of those hormones still around anyway so the tiny production from the adipose tissue is insignificant) excess body fat instead produces inflammatory substances which in turn contribute to accumulation of β amyloid, with β amyloid removal from the brain also being reduced as described above.

What is insulin, what does it do and what are type 1 diabetes, type 2 diabetes and insulin resistance?

Insulin is the hormone, which is in charge of keeping blood glucose levels in line.

In Type 1 diabetes, the body cells that produce insulin have been completely destroyed so none is produced and an external supply (usually delivered by injection) is needed. However, without internal sensors to register tiny fluctuations in blood glucose levels and adjust insulin dose accordingly, keeping blood glucose levels just right by balancing injected insulin with food and activity can be a challenge, as anyone with type 1 will know.

In Type 2 diabetes, insulin is still produced but the supply has become inadequate to keep blood glucose at ideal levels. There are likely many contributors to the development of type 2 diabetes, with overweight and inactivity making significant contributions in the vast majority of cases in younger and middle aged adults. Those are a part of the picture for anyone diagnosed with diabetes in their 80s and beyond – but world experts contend that insulin supply is challenged merely by living to advanced years. Advanced age considerations in type 2 diabetes are discussed in this chapter in greater detail because in these cases medical treatment may do more harm than good and thus often needs to be avoided. For those somewhat younger, there are all sorts of medical strategies available to assist in control of blood glucose levels in type 2 diabetes, including tablets and injections. Anyone who is overweight must do all they can to lose the excess, and increasing exercise and activity are essential because excess bodyweight forces the body to produce more insulin than would otherwise be required, so worsens the situation. It's thought that over the years supply can effectively become *exhausted*. For anyone – younger or even much older – increasing activity and exercise is the best option: exercising muscles greatly assist the actions of insulin so even when the amount available is reduced it is able to work more effectively.

Insulin resistance (IR) is a situation where there is insulin being produced in the body but for a variety of reasons the body cells that should respond to it by moving glucose from the blood into the cells where it is needed, fail to do so as well as they should. The result is that the body needs to produce more insulin than is normal and that has a range of health consequences, including probably contributing to dementia as discussed in this chapter. This forced extra insulin production usually keeps blood glucose at apparently *normal* levels for quite some time so simple blood glucose tests don't tend to detect IR. Nevertheless, anyone who is overweight in young adulthood or middle age or leads an inactive life is at risk. Obesity can be a sign of hidden IR in fact because insulin plays a part in increasing body fat stores so that higher insulin production can contribute to excess weight gain, creating a vicious cycle of weight gain and worsening IR in younger and middle aged adults especially. Fortunately, IR is usually effectively countered by activity and exercise in the same way as type 2 diabetes: increasing activity and exercise reduces insulin resistance and assists insulin action throughout the body (and brain). That's important because, left unchecked IR can progress to type 2 diabetes in time as the overproduction of insulin eventually seems to *exhaust* the supply.

In all three situations, the needs of people from their 70s on are not the same as younger adults and that must be acknowledged and considered in advice to avoid causing more harm than good. One thing remains absolutely clear – no matter how old, exercise and activity are key to reducing the effects of diabetes and IR on the brain.

Will weight loss help me avoid cognitive issues and dementia?

The short answer is yes, but it must happen before you reach later age. Of course, there are no guarantees but everything we know so far supports what has been said repeatedly in this book and in *Eat To Cheat Ageing*: activity and exercise are undeniably essential for both body and brain health.

If you are now in your late 70s or beyond, and carrying a lot of excess weight, it is possible to address that for your brain's sake. But don't do that relying on dieting or any other sort of food restriction alone, (that includes both surgical and pharmacological weight loss strategies), because the muscle loss that will cause will make things worse: it *must* also involve very good exercise. You will certainly need professional assistance to avoid possible hypos and to make sure you preserve your muscle at the same time as losing some extra body fat.

The benefits of exercise go well beyond any chance you will lose excess weight – you may lose a bit but it's the reduction in insulin resistance that is the most useful for your brain – bringing wide ranging benefits that can only help.

Interestingly doing your exercise *after* you eat gives extra benefits in a number of ways so put that into your planning. This is especially important after the evening meal where it's all too common to sit in front of the TV or on the couch reading before you head off to bed; a walk at that time will do so much good!

The big question: 'tight control' or not: good or bad for your brain?

Eat To Cheat Ageing covers more about diabetes management generally at later age. Here I want to look more closely at how those considerations play out when it comes to cognitive decline and dementia.

Tight control in diabetes means keeping the levels of glucose in the blood close to the level of a person who doesn't have diabetes. You particularly want to avoid them being higher than normal because that is what does the damage to nerves and small blood vessels throughout the body (in the heart, kidneys, eyes and the feet) as well as affecting the brain.

But in order to avoid high levels with tight control, there is always a risk that blood glucose levels will fall below this target range now and then, causing a hypoglycaemic reaction (a *hypo*).

Now, for a younger person, the experience of a hypo is distressing but not usually dangerous. For anyone in his or her later years it most certainly can be serious. A fall can far too easily snatch away health and independence so a time will come to decide if it's better to relax diabetes control. In later old age, especially if you are frail, a hypo can also lead to stroke or a heart attack as well as being far more likely to have long-term impacts on cognition.

It is a very individual decision, and you must keep revisiting your requirements every year or so if you are living with diabetes and dementia, and more often if you are unwell, or past 80. Relaxing control to avoid the chance of a hypo will also mean blood glucose levels will rise higher than those you (and your doctor) may have been comfortable with in the past.

Relaxed control has big advantages when it comes to eating well and avoiding malnutrition. It allows greater flexibility in what you eat because you don't have to worry as much about avoiding some foods that might in the past have had your levels creeping up. It helps keep your appetite up if it's failing because you get to have a few more treats than before – always good for a fragile appetite - and lets you eat enough food to help your body confront the challenges of age.

Another reason for thinking about relaxing blood glucose control is that it reduces the completely reasonable fear of suffering a hypo. When people are worried about the harm that a fall due to a hypo can cause, they may over consume carbohydrates and thus bring about elevated blood glucose levels – relaxing control means avoiding such issues.

But relaxing control is not for everyone. If you are still in your 60s or 70s and quite well, then you have decades ahead and the benefits of tight control easily outweigh the risks of a hypo. As long as you eat according to the advice elsewhere in this book, you'll enjoy those years. You'll just need to regularly reassess how you are doing as you move into your 80s and beyond and possibly rethink employing tight control as time goes on.

The importance of exercise and how to plan for it with diabetes

Exercise is an extremely important part of diabetes management at any age and as you well know, it's great for your brain, but can also trigger hypos in some people if your exercise is not adequately planned. That's because if you are on insulin or taking certain medications, adding exercise can bring your blood glucose levels down low enough to cause a hypo. However, that's no reason at all to avoid exercise, all you need to do is add extra carbohydrate-containing snacks and drinks and, in some cases, adjust your insulin or other medication dose when you exercise. You need to discuss all this with your diabetes team to develop a plan that's best for you. It's clear that whether you have type 1 or type 2 diabetes, are lean, or overweight, exercise will improve your diabetes control, help you avoid complications and continue living the life you had hoped for.

Of course, you must always check with your doctor before you start any strenuous exercise plan, but don't allow yourself to become complacent, you might be able to achieve more than you thought you could.

Chapter 7

THE GUT-BRAIN AXIS, AND GETTING FOOD FROM THE PLATE TO THE GUT

A feeling in my gut - how what lives in your GI tract affects cognition

I know it might seem somewhat strange but what is inside your gastrointestinal tract (or more simply, your gut) has a powerful influence on your mood, behaviour, and the health of your brain.

There are an almost unimaginable one hundred trillion or so - that's 10^{14} for maths buffs among you - bacteria living in the gut: so many they are now thought of as another body organ - the gut microbiome. These many, varied bacteria are indispensable to us because they are able to harvest energy and nutrients that are otherwise unavailable from food we eat. They do so much more than that because they also produce an array of chemical messengers that are able to communicate with and influence the chemistry of the brain.

These chemical messengers do this in a number of ways: Some impact the body hormone system, so can influence appetite, mood, emotions, and reactions to stress. Some impact the production of the neurotransmitters, including serotonin and GABA (both associated more with positive emotions and calmness than stress and aggression). It's recently been found that some also help promote brain health by nurturing the glia, which support and protect brain neurones. What's really interesting is that when the variety of different types of bacteria in the gut is lower (ie: a reduced diversity) that may increase inflammation, cognitive decline and frailty, as well as obesity, because under those conditions substances called cytokines that increase inflammation are produced.

~ ~ ~

'Good' bacteria versus 'bad': how a healthy gut microbiome influences the brain

You will probably have heard discussion of 'good' versus 'bad' bacteria in the gut and its quite true that the overall health of the gut microbiome aligns with the types and diversity of bacteria that live there and the balance of the 'good' and the 'bad'. When the variety of different types of bacteria in the gut reduces, that seems to mean it's mostly the 'good' ones missing, so increasing diversity in the types of gut bacteria means encouraging more 'good guys' and less 'bad'. What's also become clear in recent years is that the health of the brain and the health of the gut microbiome are inextricably linked through a communication hub called the gut-brain axis.

The gut-brain axis influences and is influenced by the emotional and cognitive centres of the brain and this is where the system can be helpful or not so helpful. The brain affects the survival of different bacteria by changing things like the 'leakiness' of the gut wall (that allows some substances through into the blood while others are excluded), and its motility (the rate of pulsing that moves contents along through the gut). In addition, it releases chemical messengers and creates a local environment that helps some types of bacteria to thrive, and others to decline. A number of things, including a calm outlook and good stress management strategies seem to swing that balance towards the good guys while anxiety and elevated stress levels give the not so good guys a better chance.

If the balance in the microbiome is in favour of the good guys the messages going back to the brain tend to continue to also be helpful –

promoting better mood, reduced anxiety, and reduced inflammation, and as a result, better brain health.

How much we can influence this balance, is not clear yet from the research and the technologies we have available. But what we eat, as outlined below can certainly help and because our brain also has such an important role to play, anything we can do to manage stress is essential

~ ~ ~

How the brain influences the gut and its inhabitants.

Overall, lower anxiety and stress levels tend to stimulate the nerve that manages swallowing and digestion called the vagus nerve; digestion is settled, heart rate calmed, and predominantly good things like improved memory, immune function, and sleep result, as well as further reducing anxiety levels. At the same time, that reduces chronic inflammation. A healthy gut microbiome (with a high proportion of 'good' bacteria and fewer 'bad') aids and abets that tendency.

However, in those who have a greater tendency to anxiety the opposite occurs and things like heart palpitations and gastrointestinal distress become more common as well as increased inflammation and an overstimulated immune response. Perhaps as a result, or just as likely it could be the cause, the gut microbiome tends to be less 'healthy', with fewer 'good' bacteria and more 'bad.'

Another big benefit of a healthy gut microbiome is that it seems able to increase levels of the Brain Derived Neurotrophic Factor (BDNF) (check that out in Chapter 1), which is involved in brain plasticity. That means that the brain is more able to adapt and cope if damage occurs.

You are not expected to change your personality of course, but finding a way to manage anxiety is well worth the effort to help your gut as well as your brain. Activity, exercise, social interaction, laughing, and avoiding an overly sedentary lifestyle is powerful; but as well it may require the assistance of medication, psychological therapies, meditation, yoga, acupuncture, or whatever works for you.

~ ~ ~

Food for a healthy gut microbiome

When it comes to food, you can do a lot to boost the good bacteria and deter the bad.

There are three ways to do that. Firstly, encourage the growth of good bacteria already in the gut by providing nutrients that those bacteria particularly like, found in so-called pre-biotic foods. Secondly, introduce new good bacteria by taking probiotics or eating probiotic foods that contain beneficial bacteria, as listed below. Lastly, minimise foods that are thought to swing the balance of bacteria towards the bad guys. These tend to be those foods that have undergone more processing and contain high amounts of cooking fats (think battered and fried foods, commercial biscuits, cookies, commercial cakes, pies, pastries, and desserts, most so called 'fast foods,' fries, and snack foods like chips and similar, soft drinks and confectionery)

The thing about both pre- and pro- biotics is they really can't do harm and often provide all sorts of other useful nutrients as well so are definitely worth a try. But take care if you don't usually eat a lot of these prebiotic foods here because the fibre and other substances in them can create lots of wind! If you want to eat more of them, or start adding new things, do so gradually and build up- that gives the bacteria in your gut a chance to get used to the change, to adapt and for the right sorts to gradually build up and help you out.

If you already have issues with bloating and abdominal pain, then get advice before adding any of these because they are likely to make things worse.

When it comes to probiotics and probiotic foods, different companies producing these use different mixes of bacteria and some products

PREBIOTICS:

Grain foods:	wheat, oats, barley and rye and foods made from them including bread, crackers, pasta, gnocchi, couscous,
Vegetables:	chicory root (this is the root of the plant often called witlof – the leaves are not high in prebiotics), garlic, onion, leek, spring onion, shallots, asparagus, beetroot, fennel bulb, green peas, snow peas, sweet corn, savoy cabbage, Jerusalem artichokes
Legumes:	kidney beans, lentils, chickpeas, all dried beans
Fruit:	white peaches, nectarines, watermelon, persimmon, Custard apples, tamarillo, grapefruit, pomegranate (including seeds), dried fruit (especially dates and figs) green or under-ripe bananas (there is not much in ripe bananas)
Nuts/seeds:	pistachios, cashews

PROBIOTICS:

Commercial preparations with 'good bacteria' (tablets or powders)

Fermented foods:	yoghurt with live bacteria
	Kimchi*, sauerkraut*
	Naturally fermented pickles* (you need to look for these or make them yourself – these use salt rather than vinegar so if vinegar is in the ingredients they are not naturally fermented)
	lassi (fermented milk drink) and similar drinks
	tempeh*(fermented soybean curd), miso
	good sourdough bread is made using a fermentation process – it will be chewy and have the traditional sour taste if its genuine

Note: contrary to some internet sites, most cheese is not fermented unless its labelled that way

*these foods are both pre- and probiotic

are more palatable than others are, but remember these contain live bacteria and they will often require refrigeration during storage.

There are many other strategies being developed and a lot of research going on now to find the best way to achieve a healthy gut microbiome beyond using pre- and pro- biotics. That is likely to be different for different people, and might even involve a scary concept known as a faecal (or fecal) transplant. That's where gut bacteria are removed from a healthy gut, or those from a less healthy gut are 'cleaned' to end up with a high number of 'good' bacteria that are then reintroduced to swing the balance there towards the good. As they say, 'watch this space' – this is something you will hear a lot about in the next few years and beyond.

~ ~ ~

The gut-brain axis and the immune system

The gut-brain axis is essential for our protection because while food and anything we put in our mouths contains a huge array of things that are good for us, there are always going to be some that can do us harm. The gut microbiome monitors what's there, 'senses' bad things, and passes the information to the gut-brain axis, that then coordinates an immune response.

That response tends to have two 'tiers': vomiting and diarrhoea are the first line of defence for the gut, causing as rapid a removal of the offending contents as possible.

The second line of defence gets a bit more complex. The brain and the gut bacteria are able to influence the 'leakiness' of the gut wall as well as its motility.

Changes in leakiness or motility can be powerful over time: excessive motility moves contents through too quickly so valuable nutrients don't get enough time to be absorbed and excessive leakiness can allow substances to get through the gut wall that are not helpful, or that potentially are a problem.

The second line of defence swings into action bringing in its impressive array of resources when something slips through the gut wall that would not usually do so. That includes a number of substances that trigger inflammation. Inflammation is an important part of the immune response if there is a real threat because it is able to call in resources from all over the body to wherever the problem has been found to help deal with it. But the problem with the leaky gut is that this immune response happens too often and too widely, triggering autoimmune problems and chronic inflammation which potentially contributes to dementia. Not only that, but because the gut-brain axis is in play, emotions and anxiety influence, and are in turn influenced, by the process.

There is such a lot going on and we have so much more to learn about the gut-brain axis, but we know that some bacteria (the 'good') tend to help reduce excessive leakiness and dampen over-inflammation as well as potentially positively influencing emotion, anxiety, mood, and more; and in contrast there are some (the 'bad') that do the opposite.

All the things that result in a settled digestive process also reduce inflammation and are associated with improved memory and cognitive function.

A NOTE ON IBS (IRRITABLE BOWEL SYNDROME) AND PRE-BIOTIC FOODS

For reasons we are only just beginning to understand and that may well involve the gut-brain axis, some people develop an *irritable* bowel. It is excessively *leaky* and hypersensitive to components of foods that most people tolerate well. Individuals may suffer chronic diarrhoea or chronic constipation and significant abdominal pain and discomfort.

One therapy that can dramatically reduce symptoms, bringing welcome relief to those living with IBS is a scientifically researched therapeutic diet known by the acronym FODMAP. It restricts a number of foods containing substances that cause the gut bacteria to react, creating symptoms. Some of the substances restricted on this diet are pre-biotics and for people with IBS, foods containing these may not be tolerated so those with IBS shouldn't start eating those foods without professional advice.

If you have issues with IBS, it is best you discuss these with an Accredited Practising Dietitian for advice.

But there is increasing evidence that probiotics can help people with IBS so they are worth a try and shouldn't cause any worsening of IBS.

Oral health and the brain

It comes as no surprise that if you teeth and your mouth aren't as healthy as they could be you are not going to be able to eat as well as you need to.

But what is surprising is how often that is forgotten or overlooked in care.

When it comes to brain health, oral health plays an important role for two reasons.

Firstly, infections in the teeth, the structures that support them and the gums, cause inflammation that extends far from the mouth, contributing to the inflammatory damage in the brain.

What infections and disease in teeth, gums, and supporting structures (periodontal) can do in older people (apart from the obvious discomfort, pain, and cosmetic issues):

Cause:

Chronic inflammation

Poor food intake

Contribute to:

Swallowing issues,

Blood loss and resultant anaemia

Aspiration pneumonia

Secondly, poor oral health, pain, a dry mouth or ill-fitting dentures can make eating otherwise enjoyable foods difficult, so contribute to malnutrition.

In someone living with dementia in the early stages, teeth cleaning or denture maintenance may continue as usual, but many aspects of self-care can become challenging in time. It may be the coordination of the steps involved in cleaning becomes difficult, or it gets forgotten, dentures are very often lost or misplaced at home and in residential care, but also as dementia progresses if they get hidden, it may be nigh on impossible to find them at mealtime. Of course losing or misplacing dentures has a huge impact on the ability to eat.

Another issue is that those who are living with dementia may not register or be able to communicate pain or discomfort as they once did.

If someone has loose or painful teeth, if their mouth is dry, or their dentures ill fitting, they may not be able to communicate that effectively. Instead, they may refuse food, avoid things that need chewing or even in frustration, throw or hide food. There are all sorts of reasons for food refusal in dementia and for changes in preferences, but ensuring that oral health is not part of the problem is relatively easy. Clearly, any sort of food refusal or reduced intake is a potential problem in anyone with dementia so needs consideration.

In people in the later stages of dementia, too often the need for good oral care is forgotten, or is not handled very well. Encouraging tooth brushing is a good idea of course but a time will probably come when that may not be manageable. I don't know about you, but I think if someone came at me waving a toothbrush and demanding I open my mouth to have it scrubbed, I might react somewhat negatively. Oral care is incredibly important but it needs to be handled with empathy and understanding.

One thing to consider is the influence of saliva in oral health: any reduction in saliva production creates big problems in oral health as well as reducing appetite and enjoyment of food. Unfortunately, far too many medications commonly taken in later age reduce saliva production. Saliva has two main roles - firstly it moistens food so it can be chewed properly, be tasted effectively, and then formed into the right consistency to be swallowed, but secondly saliva also contains substances that help protect teeth from decay. So anything that reduces saliva production is going to reduce the chance food will be enjoyed

Medications that can cause oral health problems:

Antibiotics

Antidepressants

Antihistamines

Asthma Inhalers

Corticosteroids

Decongestants

Narcotic Pain Relievers

Statins

the same way, add to swallowing problems, and at the same time increase the chance of infection in teeth and gums. Hundreds of medications can cause these problems, including recreational drugs such as marijuana (cannabis) and cocaine. There is a list of the prescription medications here.

In a person living with dementia, a regular review of medications should always be part of the picture. In the early stages, considering changing or ceasing any might be less appropriate but as the illness progresses it is essential this happen. Quality of life and especially doing everything possible to allow a person living with dementia to enjoy every mouthful of food is essential and sometimes that will mean ceasing medications that may be creating barriers to that.

Why problems occur:

Reduced saliva flow, dehydration and poor intake of food/fluid more generally

Ill-fitting or poorly maintained dentures and resultant bacterial or fungal infection

Reduced dexterity, osteoarthritis and/or cognitive deficits that reduce cleaning efficiency or regularity

Memory issues

There are also extremely important cosmetic and social aspects to teeth, oral care, and to dentures. In someone who usually wears dentures, not having them available or not wearing them changes the way they look significantly and for many people that is understandably challenging. Also, if someone is not keeping up oral hygiene then others might react to him or her negatively with resulting distress, especially if they are not aware of the reason for the problem.

I want everyone to get the chance to enjoy every mouthful, especially anyone living with dementia, but if chewing is difficult because of teeth or denture problems, pain or inflammation, it certainly will reduce enjoyment of things previously relished like a good steak, nuts and seeds, crunchy vegetables, crisp fruits or a grainy bread.

Smelling, tasting and swallowing

Eating well involves far more than the mechanics of putting things in your mouth. Of course that's going to be far easier to achieve when food smells and tastes good and a healthy brain does so much to keep both of those up to scratch. The sense of smell is often affected in dementia and that can have all sorts of consequences, including not recognising when food is off or contributing to mistaking other things for food. The sense of taste too, can be altered, so foods once loved are rejected and unusual taste combinations come into play.

Nutrient deficiency, especially of the mineral zinc can play a part in appetite decline - read more on that in Chapter 4.

Not only that, but getting food from the plate to the gut involves an extremely complex series of coordinated actions, not the least of which is actually swallowing. In dementia the coordination of swallowing is affected, often quite early in the course of the illness, sometimes even before diagnosis.

Obviously, any problems with swallowing are going to affect nutrition but also impact the quality of life and enjoyment of food. These issues are discussed in great detail in Chapter 9 but I want to mention a couple of things here too.

There are so many small ways swallowing can go wrong so it's amazing to me that it so rarely does in people with good brain health, but in dementia and in cognitive decline where connections between nerves and muscles are disrupted or lost, it very commonly does. I've already mentioned saliva and its importance in the ability to swallow food.

~ ~ ~

Also, the vital importance of muscle in the swallowing process is under-appreciated. Muscle loss that happens with age, sedentary lifestyles, weight loss, and in dementia, affects all body muscle, including that involved in swallowing. In fact, exercise that boosts muscle activity will also boost muscle throughout the body so benefits your ability to swallow.

Most of the swallowing process is not under your control: you consciously chew and start the swallowing process, but after that, the brains' autonomic (could be called automatic) systems take over. Both the conscious and the unconscious parts of the swallow can be affected by dementia and that depends on what part of the brain is impacted.

HOW DOES SWALLOWING WORK?

It involves three phases, each of which is coordinated separately by nerve impulses in different parts of the brain. To work smoothly those nerves must instruct more than 40 different pairs of muscles to work in precisely timed sequences. It's little wonder that any hiccup in brain ability also affects swallowing.

In the first (oral) phase of a swallow, food is chewed and mixed with saliva. That's the only bit that is voluntary – you know that because it's possible to stop chewing if you wish to. Next, in the 'pharyngeal phase,' the movement of food towards the back of the mouth mostly by the tongue, triggers sensors on the palate and back of the mouth that initiate the 'oesophageal phase' where the actions of involuntary muscles along the oesophagus work in sequence to move the food 'bolus' down to the stomach.

Whether swallowing is affected and how depends on both the area of the brain impacted by dementia and the quality of the muscles in the mouth, tongue, and along the oesophagus. It's certainly clear that tongue strength can decline with age, especially in dementia. That not only impacts swallowing ability, but can be an indication of overall reduced body muscle strength.

If you have occasional issues with swallowing, it doesn't necessarily mean dementia, but it's important to have any issues checked out by a registered speech pathologist (they are experts in everything to do with speaking as well as swallowing). It is possible to use strategies to help get food down safely so it doesn't *go down the wrong way*. Read more about this fascinating area in Chapter 9.

Chapter 8

MOVE IT, MOVE IT, MOVE IT

You are tired of me saying it I know, but here I go again: there is no choice but to stay active and to do your best to get all the exercise you can for your brain's sake. That means doing both physical and mental activity woven in with a healthy dose of socialising. Continuing to engage in spirited conversation, laugh, love, and cry with family and friends, prepare and savour great meals, enjoy music and books, ride a bike, decide if a piece of art is worth the canvas it's painted on, and all the things you have to do to accomplish every day-to-day task, make life what it is. Being able to do all that while continually assessing the safety and appropriateness of everything you do; be it walking along a beach or doing the shopping, to driving a car, playing tennis, or organising a great party; all keep you on track with the people and the world around you.

Physical activity especially does a number of great things for your brain:

- it maximises blood flow to get good stuff (nutrients, fuels, and oxygen) into brain cells and move the bad stuff (such as oxidative wastes) out,

- it helps the brain produce Brain Derived Neurotrophic Factor (BDNF) that builds and supports both new and old brain cell connections (increasing brain plasticity),

- it assists with glucose metabolism and diabetes management and reduces insulin resistance,

- it greatly reduces chronic inflammation,

- it gives the whole brain a work out by bringing into play all the different systems from many areas in the brain that are needed to keep your walk, golf game, bike ride, gym or Zumba session planned and coordinated — from memories of technique, rules, strategies, and the like to managing muscles, balance systems, and all the senses needed to see, hear, and feel those activities.

~ ~ ~

Immobility, inactivity and your brain

Before getting into the basics of what sort and intensity of exercise to do, a few words on the danger of immobility. Of course, relaxation is vital for good health of all sorts, but our sedentary lives increase the inflammation you have read so much about in this book. We just have far too much inactive time available to us nowadays and it's too easy to find excuses to slump instead of sit straighter, sit when we could stand, drive when we could walk, take the lift when we could make the effort to walk up the stairs. As discussed in Chapter 3, research carried out with astronauts in zero gravity has shown that removing the influence of gravity on the body results in muscle and bone decline and increases inflammation.

I get it that no one on earth is experiencing zero gravity, but in later life, when the hormones and nerves that signal the building of muscle and bone are out of the picture, the effect of being immobile is very similar to what astronauts face. The old-fashioned 'bed rest' recommended in illness and injury needs to be kept to a minimum for your body and your brain. Sure rest when it's needed, but as soon as you can, sit up, stand up, and get out of bed: work against gravity at every opportunity. Every minute you are active or do something that makes you work against gravity helps reduce inflammation and boosts your brain. No matter what you weigh, if you spend less time watching TV, sitting at the computer or in an armchair, driving in the car or sitting on a bus and more time just being up and about, moving around, that will help your body and your brain.

Add to that exercise that pushes your muscles to boost strength and increase the benefits to body and brain.

Sure exercise may be more of a struggle when older and it's going to have your muscles complaining bitterly if you are out of practice till they get used to the idea, but that only means they are listening to the messages you are sending, that they are still loved and needed! They will help you and your brain if you help them.

Naturally, all activity at later age should be discussed with your doctor and is best done with the assistance of a qualified exercise professional.

Exercise options and strategies

You can do any sort of activity you enjoy – dance, do a group class, walk (but you will need to add in some hills or spurts of increased pace to push it), swim, ride a bike, a gym program designed especially for you is ideal – whatever it is follow these basic rules. They are general in nature but if you need more, consult an exercise physiologist, or physiotherapist, or look at the information and resources provided by the groups mentioned at the end of this chapter.

Firstly:

- always warm up and cool down for at least five minutes either side of exercise by walking or doing light movements of the muscle areas you are planning to work

and a few words of caution:

- don't exercise if you are ill. It's okay if you are recovering from an accident or surgery and are able to do some exercises, but not if you are actually suffering an illness
- build up all activity gradually
- you should expect to feel mild muscle soreness in the days after exercise but as you get used to each activity that will

fade. Any severe pain means stopping that exercise and needs to be checked with your doctor, physiotherapist, or qualified exercise professional.

Next,

Plan your exercises!

To avoid overuse causing you excess pain, use different muscle group on different days. It's best to plan to use one or two major muscle groups each time you do strength exercises especially. Then after a couple of days, work a different group. Allow at least a few days between repeating an activity in the same muscle group.

Aerobic activities like walking, jogging, cycling, swimming, and sport activities use a wide range of muscles and won't usually require these considerations, though you do have to work up the length of time you spend on each.

Resistance bands and weights

Resistance bands are flexible elasticised bands that are wrapped round your hands while you do activities to help you work against the resistance they present. Your exercise professional can instruct you how to use them.

You can purchase 500g or 1kg (1 or 2 lb) hand or ankle weights (or heavier) but you can also use everyday items such as cans of soup or even bags of shopping.

With both, it's essential to start slowly at the lowest weight you need. For some people, that may be no weight at all at first, then working up to heavier weights as you progress.

To be assured you are gaining benefit, each activity should feel challenging and even a bit hard.

The weight is too heavy if you can't repeat the exercise eight times and you should then drop back in weight until your muscles have become accustomed to the lower weight.

Aim to be able to repeat each exercise 10 to 15 times. When you can do those easily, you can add more weight if you wish and are able.

Don't move too fast and don't quickly drop your weights. A rule of thumb is to count to three as you lift, push or pull; hold for one count then take two counts to return to rest.

Always breathe out as you lift, push or pull, and breathe in as you return to rest.

~ ~ ~

You need to do physical exercise regularly: combining aerobic activities like walking or anything you do that makes you puff, with things that make your muscles work hard enough so you feel it.

Walking is usually not enough. If you play a sport, do activities such as rowing, extensive bushwalking or cycling that combine strength activity with aerobic, that is ideal. Many people will be involved in gym work, which is a good option when it combines strength work with balance and aerobic activity. 'Gentle exercises' are all some people will be able to manage and anything is better than inactivity, but these are best seen as a starting point. Build on those gentle exercises as soon as you can (ideally under the guidance of a qualified exercise professional) to gain strength and ability, to help your brain do better in other things and stem cognitive decline.

One thing I think is a worthwhile muscle and brain exercise is getting up from the floor. It's relatively easy to get down to the floor – whether you do that quickly with a thud or more gracefully. But practicing getting yourself up to standing again is a great way to boost muscle strength and thereby benefit the brain at the same time. Of course, don't do that without someone close by if you are not sure you will make it up safely! And if it's been a long time since you sat on the floor, it won't be easy at first so take it slowly, in stages till you build up strength, but the more you practice that, the stronger the muscles used to fight gravity and get you upright.

The challenge of the new, the comfort of the old

Not surprisingly, your brain also likes to learn and to be challenged by new things as much as it loves being nurtured by the familiar. So when you learn something you haven't done before — an exercise program like tai chi perhaps, new card games, a new dance step, take up a new sport or learn a new language, or when you make the effort to meet new people or practise skills that require concentration— all are doing something for your brain. They're supporting and protecting it and can even cause it to form new internal connections to keep up the pace. Combine that with keeping up with things you have always enjoyed, don't neglect your love of dancing, singing, or preparing your all-time favourite meal – mixing the nourishment of the old with the challenges of the new gives your brain the support it needs from you.

As mentioned above, never discount the vital importance of keeping up social activities. Hanging out with other people means much more to the brain than merely avoiding loneliness, it means it must continue to mastermind all the very complex thought processes involved in making conversation, behaving appropriately, negotiating, and all the other things you need to juggle in social situations.

Interestingly social connectedness, along with vigorous exercise, also helps keep levels of things like brain derived neurotrophic factor (BDNF) up – so boost your brain in more ways.

In fact, even without doing mental exercises, the people who keep up social involvement along with physical exercise have the best brain health. The added bonus of remaining socially involved, from a food point of view, is that doing things socially often includes meals or, at the very least, snacks!

BASIC GUIDELINES FOR EXERCISE FOR MUSCLE AND BRAIN FUNCTION

The ideal is to combine aerobic, resistance, flexibility, and balance activities so you need to find activities, which you are able to do, which don't put you at risk of falling and ideally, which interest you. Professional assistance is ideal but not essential. Everyday activities like vacuuming and mopping, raking, sweeping, gardening, carrying the shopping, and doing housework also contributes but any activity beyond those is great. This is a guide to the intensity you need to aim for; anything you take on to achieve them is fabulous! Dance, ride a bike, swim, head to the gym, add intensity to your daily walk by picking up the pace, or taking on some steps or hills, try out the latest exercise class – all of course as safely as possible.

Aerobic

on at least 3 days per week initially, increasing to every day

aim for 30 to 60 minutes each day, which can be accumulated in 10 minute bouts

make at least 20 or 30 minutes of this time at vigorous intensity (puffing and sweating)

Resistance

weight training on at least 2 days per week

exercises for all major muscle groups: legs, arms, abdomen, hips, back, chest, shoulders

repeat each exercise 8 to 12 times

increase the weight you lift as it gets easier or repeat more times

Flexibility

sustained stretches for each major muscle group on at least 2 days per week

use static stretches, not those involving movement

Balance

on at least 1 day and eventually up to 7 days do 4 to 10 different balance activities in a safe environment only, repeat each 1 or 2 times

There is information that is more detailed, including examples of exercises, and how to measure your exercise intensity, in the appendix of this book *Eat To Cheat Ageing*.

Chapter 9

STRATEGIES WITH FOOD WHEN YOU ARE LIVING WITH DEMENTIA

As I said in the introduction and in previous chapters, a diagnosis of dementia certainly throws up some challenges, but in no way does it mean that people will immediately cease to enjoy food as much as they always have. Some types of dementia progress quite rapidly but many do not. Connections between some parts of the brain might not be working as well as they once did, meaning the ability to communicate likes and dislikes (especially in a socially acceptable manner), or to get a meal down safely might have gone astray. But by and large, these things can all be managed with a bit of creative thinking, empathy, and most of all by considering the individual.

Every person living with dementia is different. There is no plan that will work for all, and different types of dementia may necessitate completely different strategies. I'm not going to separate advice into different diagnoses here because it's just not feasible. Everything comes down to the individual dear reader, so take what helps you, always keeping in mind that everyone deserves to maintain dignity as well as enjoyment of food.

When thinking about eating and nutrition in dementia, it is so important to remember the maze I described in Chapter 1. When it comes to food it's the moving of those walls that causes most issues: lost connections between neurones mean information is not experienced in the same way as it once was, so the process of getting from hungry to enjoying a meal can be anything from a bit of a challenge to nigh on impossible.

Things that might happen when food is presented to someone with dementia, no matter how good a cook you are:

- Straight out refusal to eat.

- Lack of any response when meal is presented.

- Walking away instead of sitting at the table.

- Refusing to sit at the table.

- Food gets pushed around the plate but doesn't make it to the mouth.

- There are issues with swallowing (covered below) that mean food is spat out, spills out of the mouth during chewing, or is chewed endlessly.

- Food is put in a pocket, slipped under the plate or put somewhere *for later* instead of being eaten.

- Familiar foods become unrecognisable, or are perceived differently, as can happen due to alterations in taste and smell.

- Cooking and/or eating utensils may not be recognised or used properly.

- Frustration at not being able to communicate likes/dislikes/ hunger or swallowing issues might cause food to be thrown or angrily pushed away.

If you care about someone with dementia, it's very hard to not take it personally when meals and lovingly prepared dishes are rejected or worse, spat out or found later in the pot plant. Try not to see it as a reflection on your skills as a kitchen god or goddess, instead think of the maze, and work around the problem.

If someone wants to eat the same thing every meal or makes unusual food choices, try to work with that by adding extra nutrition to what has been chosen. There are many suggestions here that may help. Remember, if it's frustrating for you, imagine how distressing it might be for the person living with the dementia!

Anyone dealing with mild cognitive impairment has plenty to work with from the rest of this book. For those in the early stages getting enough in to help body and brain might involve just thinking protein and colours as much as possible with a focus on adding what's needed to avoiding losing weight – the suggestions in eating Plan 1 are probably enough.

This chapter is mostly for those who are preparing food, or assisting to do that, for people living with dementia. It's impossible of course to say exactly what to eat for each person because everyone is at a different stage and everyone is different. The advice is general here and tends towards those requiring more assistance with achieving adequate nutrition. I hope you will be able to gather strategies from what's here.

~ ~ ~

What's most important?

Beyond keeping the joy in eating, helping a person living with dementia to maintain weight is the best thing that can be done.

Weight loss and associated malnutrition are common and while unfortunately are sometimes unavoidable; every little thing that can be done to keep them at bay will help maintain quality of life and dignity. Not only that, but also every mouthful eaten and every meal enjoyed wards off the resulting illness and physical decline that can so easily snatch away independence if allowed to take hold.

I wonder in fact if some of the diet strategies that people take up to try to keep dementia or its progression at bay, like adding coconut oil to lots of foods and meals or starting up with green smoothies or high protein juice/nut drinks etc., might owe some of their success to the fact they helped to avoid or minimise weight loss. I'm not suggesting at all that those strategies don't provide benefit from their MCTs, antioxidants, and anti-inflammatory components - of course, they do - but if they avoid weight loss, they have been important even without those extras.

One thing to keep in mind: If you are preparing food, or assisting with meals and snacks for someone with dementia, you may have to put aside the sorts of things you need to think about when it comes to your own diet. Certainly, you have to look after yourself as well as those you care about, but their needs are unique and you mustn't confuse them with yours.

What I mean is that *you* might need to watch your calories/kJ and keep off the fatty foods, but they probably don't. You would be well advised to look at *Eat To Cheat Ageing* for some help with keeping you hale and hearty. However, for people with dementia, given their higher energy needs (as discussed in Chapter 5) most will eventually face weight loss and inadequate nutrition, so providing higher calorie/kJ foods is essential. That means helping those with dementia embrace cream, butter, and full cream milk, enjoy a bit more fat on meat, get into the fried fish and chips, and use plenty of good oil and proper (not reduced fat) mayonnaise made with oil.

Suggestions for ways to boost calories/kJ and nutrients are in the eating advice in the next chapter.

A FEW EASY THINGS TO REMEMBER TO HELP ACHIEVE GOOD FOOD INTAKE IN DEMENTIA

Pick and choose what you think might help – these are not all essential for all people

If you are caring for someone with dementia, involve him or her in meal preparation if possible.

De-clutter the table or eating space (clutter increases confusion).

Set up an eating space that ideally is used for nothing else, or if that's not possible, set the table the same way at each mealtime.

As often as possible, keep mealtimes predictable and routine and allow plenty of time.

Good lighting without glare is important (the lights will most probably be brighter than you would wish – candles alone will more likely confuse things, especially if they flicker).

Set the table so there is as much differentiation between the table and the plate and between the plate and the food as possible. Use coloured plates and contrasting tablecloth (or no tablecloth is sometimes better if possible to avoid mishaps if the tablecloth can slip). Most food has better contrast on a coloured plate. Avoid patterned plates as they increase confusion and so food gets 'lost.'

Avoid noisy, busy environments for meals. If you do go to a family event or a gathering, where it will be noisy or distracting, don't fret over food. Accept that nothing much may be eaten, or just offer known, liked foods (often sweet things work well). One meal won't matter; you can always try for a better food intake when you are home again.

Reduce choice in food offered and avoid asking about food preferences to reduce the need for decision making if that's an issue.

Even if you are not planning to eat with the person who has dementia, sit down with them as they eat and have a cup of tea or something. Evidence shows most people eat far better when they have company at the table.

Keep food expected to be hot that way and food expected to be cold that way too. This reduces confusion.

If you need to determine preference for foods, pictures will be a great help

There are all sorts of modified cutlery and crockery that can help – there are places listed to find those in the last chapter.

First, an important consideration: the big issues in swallowing.

Swallowing is a very complex process involving lots and lots of nerve connections and it can be affected from early on in dementia and even during mild cognitive impairment. The process is described in more detail in Chapter 7.

Swallowing problems are more likely in people who have lost weight and body muscle and worsen if that continues, but they can be reduced and possibly even reversed in the earlier stages if people get good exercise and rebuild muscle strength.

The sorts of things that you might see if things have gone wrong:

- Bits of food spill out of from the mouth during chewing
- Chewing goes on and on but food isn't swallowed
- Food is spat out
- Food is held in the mouth without being chewed or swallowed
- Food keeps being added to the mouth even though what's there hasn't been chewed/swallowed
- There is coughing or throat clearing during or straight after eating
- You hear gurgling or a changed voice (*wet* sounding) straight after eating or drinking.

All these things need the advice of a speech pathologist/therapist (or speech-language-therapist), ideally someone experienced in aged care and dementia.

One strategy that is instigated when there are difficulties especially with swallowing liquids is the thickening of all fluids (adding thickener to drinks or liquid foods to give them the texture of honey or custard or even thicker). As well, many foods are restricted because they are crumbly or dry. The reasoning behind this is that inefficient or inadequate swallowing accidentally delivers liquids or crumbs of food into the lungs instead of the stomach where it sets up an infection, leading to potentially fatal pneumonia. This is called aspiration and the reasoning is that if fluids are 'thicker' and foods less dry and crumbly there is less chance little bits will get into the wrong place.

There are three main issues to consider here:

Firstly, does this work to stop pneumonia?

Well, overall the answer would be yes. But there has been research done that shows the automatic thickening of liquids and avoidance of crumbly foods might need to be re-evaluated in some situations. Yes, of course, food getting into the lungs is a problem but there is far more to developing an infection as a result of that than eating toast or drinking water straight from the tap.

Researchers suggest there needs to be a greater emphasis on looking at the wider picture. Things that should be added into the mix include: was the individual being tested fully awake at the time? This might seem to be an obvious consideration, but it's amazing how frequently it's not. It might depend on the time of day, on whether there is an infection or other illness in the picture, or very frequently on the medications that might be being taken that affect alertness. Swallowing is far less effective if someone is not completely alert and that is extra important in dementia when the coordination may be just a little out anyway.

Other things for that mix include assisting with oral hygiene so bits of food are not left behind after eating to be accidentally inhaled later. As well, making sure the eating environment is not full of distractions and confusion allows a better focus on getting food and drink down.

These are things to discuss with the speech pathologist or speech-language-therapist.

That brings me to a second issue, the matter of informed choice:

I believe that every individual has the right to eat the food they enjoy most and that is extra important as they approach the end of their life. We take risks throughout our lives, big and small – it is our right to make the choice to do that even when we are assisted in daily living by others.

In dementia a time will come when eating and swallowing problems become so severe that it is clear that person has entered the final stages of their illness and no matter how much those who care about them would love them to stay, sadly, this is the time to consider their end of life plan.

Families naturally often ask residential aged care staff and medical practitioners to 'do something.' Feeding tubes are often proposed and sometimes used, but unfortunately, they don't prolong life significantly and in fact can also contribute to aspiration. In addition, they certainly don't improve the dignity or quality of life in most situations.

It's never an easy discussion to have and there is nothing easy about the lot of someone living with dementia, their family or friends who feel helpless in the face of this illness, but ensuring respect and dignified treatment at the end of their life is a gift anyone can aspire to provide. Having discussions early on in the illness, even though those will be challenging, is so important.

The final consideration, but the one that should be first and foremost, is, "Will thickening liquids or changing the texture of foods help maintain good food intake?" The answer is far too often, no.

Removing loved foods like toast, crumbly scones, ice cream, or a good cup of tea, or changing them with thickeners and gels, no matter how good the final product is, can just mean people won't eat them. There is no point going to the time and effort of thickening every liquid that passes the lips or stopping the supply of toast or potato crisps if the modified foods are only rejected and food/drink intake falls. By now, you know how damaging malnutrition can be.

It's a matter of taking a sensible, considered approach. Discussions about end of life and acute care should happen between the person living with dementia and their family early on in the illness to ensure dignity while balancing concerns about safety and nutrition.

So having said all that, there are plenty of options available when swallowing difficulties are apparent and an individual is content with the modified foods. There are resources listed at the end of the book, which provide recipes and advice to help. In recent years there have been wonderful advances made into preparing and developing recipes for familiar foods that are swallowing-safe. These can be made at home or in residential care and allow people living with dementia to continue to enjoy foods and drinks without losing the pleasure of eating. It all depends on the individual.

~ ~ ~

Being spoon fed – the good and the bad

People with dementia will need assistance with eating at some stage in the progression of the illness – that may range from something as simple as the set up of the eating environment as in the box here, to being provided finger food, and finally to being fed by spoon.

Many people will find 'full assistance' (being fed with a spoon) and even partial assistance, which might involve helping set up a meal in bed, opening packets, and putting on what is effectively an adult 'bib', very belittling and will react against it. Of course, full assistance may be necessary later in the progression of dementia and a gentle, considered assistance is essential. Avoid rushing in to the room poking a spoon at someone who is often already a bit confused and disoriented, that is just unlikely to go well.

~ ~ ~

Strategies to assist with eating

From early on, there are all sorts of ways people with dementia can be assisted in eating without it being demeaning. Here are some ideas to go with the strategies suggested in the box:

- Stay calm. I know that is sometimes nigh on impossible but always try to 'fake it till you make it' – if you are agitated it's pretty likely to set the meal up for problems.

- Wherever possible make food preparation visible so it's obvious a meal is on the way. If you are preparing food for a later meal then either have nutritious snacks available while you are doing that to keep up the association between food preparations and eating, or prepare the meal ahead at the same time as the current meal. That way you avoid preparing food without the immediate eating connection, which is what can otherwise make things confusing for someone with dementia.

- Prompting, demonstration (eating together so that actions can be mimicked) or gentle reminders all help.

- One idea, if there are family or friends around who share meals, is to arrange with them that they will get reminders about how to eat or what food is in front of them if it looks like the person with dementia is experiencing confusion with eating. That way mimicry is possible without embarrassment.

- Organise things so someone who has always cooked can continue to do that if possible or find ways to involve them in the meal preparation.

- Sometimes starting the meal with a 'treat' food, – often something sweet – can trigger hunger and mean that more of the meal is then eaten. This might mean having a small amount of the 'treat' available during the final stages of the meal preparation rather than on the table so it is snacked on beforehand.

- If 'regular' foods are rejected, follow the strategies below – it doesn't really matter if someone won't eat meat and three veg but will enjoy a dessert as long as the dessert is constructed with extra nutrition.

- If there are any problems, even small, with getting food down, make sure to provide soft, moist foods like casseroles, to add plenty of cream, ice cream, or custard to desserts and to use stewed or canned fruits etc. Cutting things like toast into small pieces can help.

~ ~ ~

A few things that might crop up and what you can do about them

Food stockpiling or hoarding:

This is common and is actually possibly a sign of hunger. The problem with it, apart from issues around food being stuffed behind the couch or in the bedside table drawer, is that the food rarely gets eaten and if it does, it might be off by the time that happens.

The only way to really avoid this is to 'supervise' at mealtimes. Situations vary: in some, it might be best to allow left over food to be whisked away into a hiding place from which a caretaker can surreptitiously remove it later. This will only work if hiding places are known and as long as enough (or as much as possible) has been eaten at the meal.

Mostly, sharing a meal or being around while its being eaten will help avoid this happening. Doing the things suggested above like prompting or demonstrating eating will help food go into the mouth instead of the pocket and relieve hunger, thus possibly reducing the likelihood stockpiling will happen.

It is worth considering putting locks on food cupboards if this becomes a significant non-mealtime issue. These should be locks that are not visible ideally (the sort used to keep toddlers out of cupboards work well often) to avoid them becoming a challenge to be dealt with or a source of suspicion. A good idea is to leave one or two cupboards able to be opened and in them put things you would like to see eaten. You could even put a sandwich cut into quarters or other snacks like cubes of cheese or dried fruits in there. You will have to replace them now and then of course, but they just might get eaten and if they do get added to the stockpile, as long as you know where that is, you can gather it up later.

Remember, if it is a sign of hunger the best idea is to do all you can to get enough in to relieve that – try some of the high protein drink recipes in the next chapter, or use the 'sweet treat to get the meal going' strategy.

~ ~ ~

Food safety

If someone is living independently with dementia, one thing those who care about that person can do is find a way to check, or help that person to check, that the food eaten is safe. So many hospital admissions for gastrointestinal upset in people with cognitive impairment are probably a result of food poisoning and it's so important that is avoided.

The sense of smell is very often reduced, even in the early stages of dementia and as a consequence, 'off smells' are easily missed. Food can be festering away at the back of the fridge and still be pulled out to be eaten without any concern at all. On the other hand, things that should be in the fridge can be left on the bench, incorrectly put away in a cupboard or the like.

Doing a check without causing upset and certainly without admonishment is a great idea. This might need to be done with the person who has dementia, or might be best done without them when they are out or engaged in something else. It might involve swapping old for new of the same food.

~ ~ ~

Paranoia about food

Another thing that happens in many people living with dementia is developing paranoia. This can relate to food and especially to a belief that someone is trying to poison them. This is very scary for the person in that situation and distressing for those who care about them.

It might be possible to guide food preparation allowing the person with dementia to do all the hands-on work so they don't feel there is an opportunity for food to have been contaminated, but that is not always enough.

If the concern relates to a particular food then that can be quite easily substituted, but if it is more than that professional help is best.

Any sort of paranoia really needs the guidance of dementia support services, so accessing their advice is essential.

~ ~ ~

Eating unusual things

In the behavioural type of frontotemporal dementia (FTD) and occasionally in other dementias, it is possible that things that are not food are mistaken for food. This can be anything from mildly annoying to very dangerous depending on what has been eaten.

In someone with FTD, it's always worth considering this if a gastrointestinal upset occurs, so that the doctor or hospital might have an idea what they are dealing with.

The best plan is to organise cupboard locks as suggested above for those who stockpile or hoard food to secure dangerous substances like dishwasher power and tablets, bleach and other cleaners, nail polish and polish removers, paints, and nasty things in the shed or garage. Go around your house if this is an issue and check cupboards and drawers, you can be amazed what is there.

~ ~ ~

Dealing with food memory

In people with memory impairment, especially if it's short-term memory that is reduced, the ability to recognise 'new' foods can be a challenge. Food from decades earlier might be enjoyed, even from childhood – think baked custard, stewed apple, stews, lambs fry, basic meat with three vegetables. These things are often far more easily recognised than a stir-fry with crunchy vegetables or a sushi roll which might be completely ignored even if the person is hungry. Also, even though some more old fashioned meats like lambs fry or rabbit, or older style desserts are having a bit of a comeback in trendy circles nowadays, a deconstructed lemon meringue pie, or rabbit jointed and served four ways is likely to be completely ignored if it doesn't look like the memory suggests it should.

There are so many ways eating can be impacted. Keep an open mind and if you are new to assisting a particular person living with dementia, get to know them. Ask them what they like if they are able to tell you, using pictures of food can help if this is difficult. Ask their family, friends, neighbours. Put yourself in their place and think up strategies to try.

Above all, take things slowly, don't be impatient, and spend time. Food provides so much enjoyment in life, be sure to always keep that in mind even if the person you care about doesn't appear to appreciate their meal – they just may be unable to tell you.

Chapter 10

EATING PLANS FOR LIVING WITH DEMENTIA

Everything that has been said throughout this book, especially in the last chapter, applies here. And always keep in mind that this book is all about living well with dementia. Enjoy every mouthful.

Plan 1

A BASIC PLAN FOR SOMEONE LIVING QUITE WELL WITH DEMENTIA BUT NEEDING GUIDANCE AND SUPPORT TO AVOID WEIGHT LOSS

This is designed to provide extra kilojoules as well as the protein and other nutrients needed. For the smaller number of people with frontotemporal dementia who often overeat at least in the early stages this may not be the best option, but remember that even in FTD eventually weight loss becomes an issue. The best strategy is keeping up activity in the early stages as much as possible to head off large increases. Later on, this plan or the finger food and snacks options next will apply as they do for others.

There is no need to choose low fat foods. Buy full cream milk (it's only three to four percent fat anyway), yoghurt, and dairy foods, trim your meat only of thick layers of fat, choose a quality oil, or margarine, or enjoy butter. Enjoy fish and chips, and some treat foods. Keep milk powder or a high protein supplement in the pantry to make high protein milk, yoghurt, and soups, etc.

Aim for three good meals a day, or three smaller meals with snacks between. The aim is keeping weight stable but if weight loss is an issue, add options from the next plan.

During illness or if full meals are just too much, eat desserts or have soups or smoothies instead *as long as they are high protein*. You can have six to eight good snacks a day instead of meals. It doesn't matter which choice you make as long as they give you what you need.

In addition, keep thinking of ways to add extra colour to your meals or snacks – whatever vegetables you can manage, different fruits, and herbs.

Breakfast

(Foods with asterisk have recipes at the end of this chapter.)

Cereal or porridge with high protein* (full cream) milk.

Eggs cooked any way you like them with toast and bacon or other accompaniment. Spread toast thickly with butter or an alternative spread. If you scramble eggs, use the recipe for high energy scrambled egg*.

Fruit smoothies or milkshake made from the high protein drinks* (see recipe list).

Bacon, ham or other meat with any accompaniment.

Baked beans or similar on toast. Enjoy your butter spread thickly.

Cheese on toast — use thick cheese slices on wholegrain or wholemeal bread, with tomato or other herbs or vegetables as desired.

Fruit with high protein yoghurt (mix in a dessertspoon of skim milk powder).

Main Meals

Meat, fish, seafood, chicken, egg, or other animal protein.

OR vegetarian protein food (pulses, soybeans or soy based product, nuts, seeds, quinoa).

WITH any vegetable, salad or fruit accompaniment and rice or grain food.

Pasta, rice, or bread may be added to any choice.

If it is a struggle to eat enough to get the protein needed, boost what's in each meal or mouthful. Sprinkle a little cheese or chopped ham slices over vegetables, or add cheese or nuts (not with anyone at risk of aspiration – use nut butters or satay sauce instead) to a salad, melt butter over hot vegetables for extra kilojoules, add cheese sauce* to dishes, or add high-energy gravy* to meats (see recipes).

Use high protein drinks* either between meals or as alternatives to meals if necessary. Choose a commercial supplement or make one from the recipes here.

Add a dessert. If you have had a good protein food in your main meal then dessert can be anything you fancy. But if you were not able to eat a good main meal then you can use dessert to supply your protein. Choose a high protein dessert from the recipe section.

Snacks

Snacks are useful in this plan if you are not able to eat well at each meal. If you have eaten a good protein food and a good variety of antioxidant and other foods at your meals, then snacks may not be essential. If you haven't been able to do so, and especially if you are still struggling to keep your weight up, snacks are important. The list here gives suggestions, and there are many foods in the next plan.

SNACKS

Higher protein options

Yoghurt, custard, or similar dairy snack.

Cheese and crackers.

Nuts (or nuts and dried fruit) or nut butters on bread/crackers.

Fruit with cheese.

Sliced meats.

Cakes, biscuits, snack bars with fruit, nuts, or seeds added.

Antioxidant options:

Fruit or dried fruit, fruit juice, or fruit and vegetable juice.

Biscuits, cakes, with fruits and nuts.

Fruit toast.

Smoothies made with fruit, nuts, and milk or soymilk.

Plan 2

FOR THOSE WHO HAVE LOST WEIGHT OR WHO ARE STRUGGLING TO EAT *MEALS*

I haven't divided this list into meals because any food from the suggestions is fine. Six to eight small portions of any food here is ideal and having them every 2 -3 hours is good.

Some people may be unable to sit at the table for long enough to eat a 'meal' so these snacks are a good option. Either sit down together every couple of hours or so for a snack, or put plates of finger foods from this list around the house now and then (replacing them often) so they might be picked up when passing.

First, it's a good idea to stock your pantry or fridge with items from the shopping list.

Plan 2 shopping list

High protein supplement powders	There are many varieties on the market – most are dairy based but varieties based on soy or alternatives are also available. Check chemists and chemist outlets. The supermarket brands generally don't contain the same range of nutrients. There are two Australian made products: *Enprocal* powder, a neutral flavour for sweet or savoury foods; and *Proform*, available in neutral, vanilla and chocolate. *Sustagen (Nestle), Fortisip (Nutricia)* and *Ensure (Abbott)* are the most commonly known alternatives. *Sustagen* is available now in neutral as well as the better-known vanilla and chocolate flavours, *Fortisip* and *Ensure* are vanilla flavoured and *Ensure* is the only one of these that is lactose free.
Whey based powders	Whey is a by-product of cheese production and has been shown to be especially good at improving muscle function in older people. Whey protein isolate, which is the most concentrated type, is quite costly and these powders don't have other vitamins and minerals added as those above do. But many people have found them to be especially beneficial.
Bodybuilding powders	Sold in gyms and health food stores but it's best to check with a doctor or dietitian first to be sure they are OK for you.

Milk powder or skim milk powder	These can be substituted for the protein powders (see above). They cost less but don't contain the range of nutrients that the more popular commercial supplements do. Full cream milk powder is not as high in protein as skim milk powder but has extra calories. It also imparts a richer flavour — either is suitable.
Cheese: cheddar or soft cheeses of any variety	Ready sliced, cubed, or grated cheese, packaged wedges, small portions, or cheese sticks (often used for kids' school lunches) are useful to have on hand.
Sliced meats or barbecued chicken	Store these in the fridge immediately and throw out any not used after 48 hours.
Ready-to-heat frozen snack foods	Suggestions include party pies, sausage rolls, chicken drumettes, or nuggets, mini quiches, fish cocktails and fish pieces, fish-in sauce. (frozen and cooked).
Ready-made meals:	Try to *avoid* low fat and 'diet' varieties (but, if you do buy these, add grated cheese, cream, butter or high protein gravy during reheating to boost their kilojoules), pies, and quiches.
Gravy powder or ready-made gravy and sauces	Have on hand to make up adding a protein powder.
Yoghurt: preferably NOT low fat	You need to look for any that are made using full cream milk, the ones that *don't* claim to be low fat. Some of the gourmet yoghurts are made with full cream milk as are most Greek-style yoghurts.
Other dairy desserts: custards, mousse, crème caramel, mini ice creams	*Avoid* low fat if possible, but you can always add cream at home.
Cream	Fresh or buy UHT cream to store in the pantry.
Paté	Those made from chicken liver, meat, or smoked fish.
Ice cream	The best are gourmet ice creams, which are usually higher in fat but any will do.
Canned or microwaveable dessert puddings	
Soups of any variety including Cup-of-Soup	Any sort will do but need to be prepared as below.

Small cans of tuna, salmon or any sort of meat (chicken is now also widely available).	
Small cans of baked beans	Baked beans are higher in protein than canned spaghetti.

Meal or snack options

Choose at least six to eight per day. Some of these are *finger foods* that can be eaten easily by those who are up and about most of the time.

Commercial supplement drink	Made to directions on can/packet.
Milkshake or smoothie	From recipes*.
High protein fruit, vegetable juice or fruit and vegetable smoothie	From recipes*.
Iced coffee with or without sweetening	From recipes*.
High protein yoghurt	Yoghurt or custard with a heaped dessertspoon of high protein supplement powder (neutral flavour or vanilla) or milk powder added.
Fruit with high protein yoghurt	
Cup-of-Soup (or pre-made soup)	With one or two heaped dessertspoons of high protein supplement (neutral) or milk powder added.
Any of your frozen snack foods	Reheated and put on a plate with tomato sauce or the usual accompaniments.
Scrambled egg or boiled egg	Hard-boiled egg with mayonnaise is another good option.
Egg, cheese or meat sandwich	With salad if you prefer.
Toasted sandwich with cheese alone or with baked beans, sweet corn, tomato, or meat	Cut into quarters as a finger food.
Cheese with crackers or sticks of celery, carrot or apple	Use meat and salad with some cheese.
Mini burgers using small buns	

Paté and crackers or toast	
Peanut butter on toast	
Cheese or baked beans on toast	
Ice cream	With a heaped spoonful of a flavoured high protein supplement powder (vanilla or chocolate) or sprinkled with chocolate drink powder (*Milo, Ovaltine, Akta-Vite,* etc.)
Handful of nuts, or nuts and dried fruit	(if aspiration is not an issue.)
A couple of slices of cold meat or a piece of cold barbecued chicken	
A big spoonful of peanut butter	Right from the jar if you like or fill a celery stick.
Commercial ready-made meal	If they are diet or low fat meals, add cheese for extra protein and cream for calories.
Breakfast cereal or porridge	With a heaped spoonful of a vanilla or other flavoured high protein supplement powder sprinkled over.
Any vegetable or meat with gravy, cheese, or mornay sauce	Make gravy mixes or sauce adding in a dessertspoon of protein powder of any type per serving. Or use recipes below.
A small can of tuna, salmon, or chicken	
Commercial snack bars based on nuts or marketed as high protein	These are good emergency options but avoid any that are low fat or sugar free.

There are many more finger food suggestions in recipe books listed in Chapter 11.

Sandwich Tips

- There is *no* need to avoid butter or margarine. You may put a generous spread on your bread.

- In place of butter or margarine, or even in addition, use cream cheese, cheese spread to boost the protein content of your sandwich or a good mayonnaise that is *not* low fat or reduced fat to boost kilojoules (calories).

- If a whole sandwich is too much, just have one slice of bread but fill it well.

- If you are having cold meat, have at least two slices, not just one.

- Add sliced or grated cheese to as many sandwiches as you can. Salad or tomato is great but the cheese will add protein and calcium too.

- Peanut butter or other nut butters are great protein foods for sandwiches.

- If you want a sweet sandwich then have one — jam or honey is great — but spread the bread with cream cheese rather than butter to boost the protein and calcium content of your meal.

- As an indulgence, spread your bread with butter, and then sprinkle a spoonful of *Milo* or similar powdered drink on your sandwich.

Additional lists and recipes

Drinks:

For most of these recipes, you will need to add a high protein powdered supplement. This can be any one of the following, used depending on their nutritional value, cost, flavour, and your own food preferences:

Commercial brand 'complete nutrition' products:

(These all have essential vitamins, and minerals added so can be used as complete meal alternatives).

Proform, Enprocal, Sustagen, Fortisip - all available flavoured; *Proform* and *Sustagen* are also available in neutral (unsweetened and with no added flavour). All are dairy based and contain lactose.

Ensure : is vanilla flavoured and dairy based but is lactose free.

High Protein products, which are not complete nutrition

(These are high in protein but do not have added vitamins and minerals – suitable for high protein drinks and dishes but not as complete meal replacements all the time. The variety of these available is every increasing so the following list is of those most common)

Skim Milk Powder (unflavoured)

Soy milk powder (unflavoured)

Whey protein Isolate or Whey Protein Concentrate (flavoured or unflavoured)

Soy Protein Isolate or alternative products (flavoured or unflavoured)

Bodybuilding powders (check suitability with your doctor or dietitian)

Recipe Ideas:

High protein tea or coffee

Your usual cup with a dessertspoon of powdered supplement mixed in (neutral flavour is best).

High protein milk coffee (can be iced or hot):

200ml full cream milk

1 tablespoon powdered supplement (any is acceptable – vanilla flavoured)

1 teaspoon powdered instant coffee (or granulated coffee mixed with a little hot water or a shot of espresso)

Sugar or honey to taste

If you are making iced coffee add a spoon of ice cream to the bottom of the glass, or blend it in.

Fruit smoothie:

Blend:

200ml full cream milk

2 dessertspoons of any high protein powdered supplement (can be one type or a mix of two and can be vanilla or neutral flavoured)

1 banana or other piece of fruit

Sugar or honey to taste

Non dairy fruit smoothie:

Blend well:

200ml fruit juice (non citrus is best but you can experiment)

Hand full of nuts (any variety you prefer will do though some blend better than others do)

Handful of seeds also if desired (such as flax, sesame, sunflower)

Sugar or honey to taste

High protein fruit juice:

(This will become more like a smoothie than a juice)

Blend:

200ml apple or other fruit juice (citrus juices are not suitable)

2 dessertspoons of high protein powdered supplement (neutral or vanilla)

High protein cup of soup

Use any variety of 'Cup of Soup' (best with those not usually clear soups but works with any)

Add 1-2 dessertspoons neutral flavoured high protein supplement

Make according to directions

Sauces and gravies

High protein gravy

Add 1 dessertspoon of neutral flavoured high protein powdered supplement for each serving of gravy made.

Quick cheese sauce:

1 small jar of commercial cheddar cheese spread

200ml cream

Mix while melting together slowly on the stove or microwave in 10 second bursts till a smooth sauce results

Mornay sauce:

1 cup high protein milk (or full cream milk plus 2 tablespoons neutral flavoured high protein powdered supplement)

2 tablespoons cornflour

¼ cup cream

Handful of grated cheese

Blend milk gradually into cornflour (start with a little milk then add the rest when the mix is smooth)

Add cream

Heat gradually on the stove till boiling, stirring continuously

Simmer for 1 minute

Remove from heat and add cheese (and chopped or dried herbs to taste) and mix till cheese melts

Custard

If you buy pre-made custard, mix 1 dessertspoon of high protein supplement powder (vanilla flavour or neutral) with a little milk to make a paste, and then mix into the custard

If you prefer to make your own then add 1 dessertspoon of high protein supplement powder (vanilla flavour or neutral) to your recipe per serving.

Other Recipes

Neutral flavoured high protein supplement powders can be added to any sweet or savoury dish: If you are making a casserole, curry, creamy pasta sauce, or similar dish you can add 1 dessertspoon for each serving of the meal. Its best added during cooking but in some cases can be added after cooking.

For mashed potato add 1 dessertspoon per serving when you add the milk before mashing.

Add a dessertspoon per serving to creamed rice and baked desserts (you can use flavoured or unflavoured for this).

Add 1 dessertspoon of high protein supplement powder or a handful of ground nuts or a handful of ground, mixed nuts, and seeds per serving to a cake mix.

~ ~ ~

A list of commercial supplements, where to get further information, and recipes is in the last chapter.

Chapter 11

RESOURCES AND PLACES TO GET HELP

You will know already of Alzheimer's organisations and associations for many other types of dementia – here is a brief list.

Alzheimer's Australia: **www.fightdementia.org.au**

Alzheimer's International: **www.alz.org**

Alzheimer's UK: **www.alz.co.uk**

Alzheimer's USA: **www.alzfdn.org**

Brain health and dementia: **www.yourbrainmatters.org.au**

For advice on management of challenging behaviour in dementia there is a Dementia Behaviour Management and Assistance Service (DBMAS) available. Ask your local Alzheimer's association or dementia advisor about this if you need help.

~ ~ ~

But I want to share some you may not know of that I believe are of immense help to anyone faced with a diagnosis of dementia in themselves or someone they care about.

Kate Swaffer

Kate Swaffer is a remarkable woman diagnosed with a somewhat unusual type of younger onset dementia. Her website contains a wealth of fabulous information and her blog is refreshing, honest, and insightful. It is so helpful for me as a practitioner to read Kate's blog posts and get just a glimpse into how she manages her busy, active life. I have often been guided by her posts and information on her website and I know it is helpful to anyone with even a slight interest in dementia.

She also undertook a project in 2013 to produce a recipe a day for 365 days! Remarkable! The recipes are varied and delicious and I urge you to check them out. **www.kateswaffer.com**

Maggie Beer Foundation

Maggie Beer is an inspiration and a friend and her foundation is doing great things towards making aged care 'sexy.' Of course, dementia is not all about aged care, but what the Maggie Beer Foundation is doing in aged care is fuelling a revolution in thinking in aged care food and that includes for those living with dementia.

Keep up to date with what Maggie and her team are up to here: **www.maggiebeerfoundation.org.au**

Don't Give Me Eggs That Bounce

This great book was released in 2014 – it provides excellent information for people living with dementia and those who care for and about them, as well as more than 100 recipes. Many recipes are also texture-modified versions (so are safe when there are problems with coordinating swallowing).

Chef Peter Morgan Jones has taken his skills as a master chef, listened to the needs of the people he is cooking for, as well as his dietitian, speech pathologist, and occupational therapist advisors, and devised foods that are enjoyable, and support nutrition.

At the time of producing this book Peter and his team were well into production of a follow up book to this one so look out for it also.

Some places to find excellent information about exercise

This is a great resource from Alzheimer's Australia that applies to all types of dementia:

www.fightdementia.org.au/sites/default/files/YBMPaper36_webfinal.pdf

Other resources that are also good can be found at

The Canadian Centre for Ageing and Activity Facebook page: www.facebook.com/actage

www.alzheimers.org.uk/site/scripts/documents_info.php?documentID=1764

www.yourbrainmatters.org.au/physical-activity-and-dementia-risk-%E2%80%93-evidence

And look too at *Active Ageing Australia*, an excellent group in South Australia who have resources and training programs you can access.

www.activeageingaustralia.com.au

~ ~ ~

Some interesting blogs and web pages to check out

The American Speech-Language-Hearing Association has an interesting online magazine at: www.leader.pubs.asha.org and a great blog at: www.blog.asha.org The article in the October 2015 magazine, called *Stepping Up to The Plate* is interesting: www.leader.pubs.asha.org/issue.aspx?issueid=934556#issueid=934556

And I love this brain blog – it was started in 2005 as part of the *Global Neuroscience Initiative Foundation* so it's peppered with a bit of scientific language but if you are OK with that I recommend it to keep up with reputable work being done in this area: www.brainblogger.com

These are only a couple of course, but there is plenty of rubbish on the internet so it's worth knowing a few places to go for what's based in good research.

Index

C

D

Printed in the USA
CPSIA information can be obtained
at www.ICGtesting.com
LVHW061550280923
759398LV00038B/386

9 780994 344038